Dr. C. Norman Shealy is the founder of the American Holistic Medicine Association and a world-renowned neurosurgeon. He has written many books, including the bestselling *The Self-Healing Workbook,* published by Element.

by the same author

The Creation of Health
The Pain Game
The Self-Healing Workbook

Special Note from the Publisher

This book is intended for information and guidance only. It is not intended to replace professional advice, and readers are strongly urged to consult an experienced practitioner for a proper diagnosis or assessment before trying any of the treatments outlined.

Miracles Do Happen

A Physician's Experience with Alternative Medicine

C. Norman Shealy, M.D., Ph.D.

ELEMENT

Rockport, Massachusetts • Shaftesbury, Dorset •
Brisbane, Queensland

© copyright C. Norman Shealy 1995
First published in the USA in 1995 by
Element Books, Inc.
PO Box 830, Rockport, MA 01966

Published in Great Britain in 1995 by
Element Books Limited
Shaftesbury, Dorset SP7 8BP

Published in Australia in 1995 by
Element Books Limited
for Jacaranda Wiley Limited
33 Park Road, Milton, Brisbane 4064

Cover design by the Bridgewater Book Company
Edited by Lynn Alden Kendall
Designed and typeset by Wordweaver, Inc.
Printed and bound in the USA by Edwards Brothers Inc.
British Library Cataloguing in Publication data available
Library of Congress Cataloging in Publication data available

ISBN 1-85230-688-2

Acknowledgments

The most important contributors to this book have been my friends, family, patients, clients, and students who have presented me with the opportunity to observe many different miracles. As always, there is my wonderful staff, without whom I could not get any book completed. Jody Trotter has typed and retyped and retyped this particular one, and Susan Robords has assisted greatly with the proofreading.

This book is dedicated to

the source of all miracles,

the Universal Power

that sometimes grants grace

Contents

PART ONE

Expect a Miracle

Chapter 1

Expect a Miracle

People who don't believe
in miracles aren't realists.
−Ashley Montague

Miracles transcend the body.
They are sudden shifts
into invisibility away from the bodily level.
That is why they heal.
−*A Course in Miracles*

Miracles are natural signs of
forgiveness. Through miracles
you accept God's forgiveness
by extending it to others.
−*A Course in Miracles*

Throughout history most illnesses have been treated with "folk medicine." Indeed, until the 1940s individuals were often better served if they avoided physicians or hospitals.

Then the explosion of modern technological medicine began, with introduction of a never-ending array of diagnostic and therapeutic miracles: antibiotics, tranquilizers, remarkably complex surgery, CT scans, MRI, and so on. These changes have given us the most successful medical system in history—for treatment of acute illness. Unfortunately, the glamor of these innovations has obscured the lack of attention to chronic illness. And nowhere is this deficit more obvious than in the management of depression, the most common illness in the world and the most poorly treated. In fact, tranquilizers are the most iatrogenically misused prescription drug, with antidepressants a close second. And chronic use of tranquilizers converts anxiety to depression!

Actually, however, a vast majority of illnesses are still treated not by physicians but in the folk and alternative domain. A landmark article in *The New England Journal of Medicine* proved that Americans made more visits to alternative practitioners than they made to primary physicians. And Americans spent more out of pocket on alternative therapy than they spent out of pocket for hospitalization. These figures emphasize the powerful drive to avoid medical/surgical treatment when that is the only offering of the medical profession.[1]

In the past twenty-five years, I have lectured to many thousands of Americans eager for information on self-care. Trained at the Massachusetts General Hospital in neurosurgery, I soon realized that drugs and surgery are inappropriate in the management of chronic pain, which represents about a third of the complaints of patients seen by neurosurgeons. I introduced two important techniques for pain control: dorsal column stimulation, a "pacemaker" of the spinal cord, and transcutaneous electrical nerve stimulation (TENS), now used worldwide but originally an alternative in the true sense. Even today it is used for less than 10% of patients for whom it could be helpful without significant complications; this cannot be said for any drug or surgery.

Beginning in the 1960s Humanistic Psychology introduced the concept of self-actualization, the potential for attaining a sense of personal autonomy and self-control–concepts previously reserved for the highly religious discipline of mysticism. Books proliferated, and experiential workshops enticed millions to begin a journey of personal responsibility for thoughts, actions, and ultimately for health. To some extent the Humanistic Psychology movement, spurred by the Establishment, has led the wave of alternative practices that have now culminated in the establishment by Congress of a Department of Alternative Medicine. Unfortunately, as is typical of government, this department gives no more than lip service to the concept. With its small budget and bureaucratic hassle, it is unlikely to unravel even the most superficial aspect of alternatives. Meanwhile, a few physicians have brought some aspects of alternative technology to the attention of the public. I have been one of those physicians.

In 1978 I founded the American Holistic Medical Association, and I was instrumental in promoting the beginning of the American Holistic Nurses' Association. I have published several self-help books, I do dozens of workshops and lectures each year, and I have a popular weekly call-in radio health show. Even by conservative estimates, I believe I have experienced and evaluated more alternative approaches than any other physician.

It is time to bring the vast field of alternatives into some semblance of order, to alert Americans to the benefits and the shortcomings of alternatives. I propose to give you an overview of the field of alternatives, suggestions for situations in which alternatives should be considered, and a personal judgment concerning the quality of the most common alternatives, as well as options worth considering for the most common ailments.

Many of the alternatives have produced miraculous cures that could not be expected from conventional medicine. Lest you think I am trivializing miracles as you read this account, consider this dictionary definition for the word miracle: "An event that seems inexplicable by the laws of nature."[2]

I consider any event or experience that transcends expectation, logic, or "facts" as we believe them, and that provides a numinous life change, to be a miracle. To conventional physicians and scientists, there is no white crow and thus no miracles. Such physicians reject out of hand techniques like spiritual healing, acupuncture, chiropractic, and homeopathy, and they even malign the placebo, the latter being the most potent healing force known. They reject anything that is inexplicable by their own perceived "laws."

And yet virtually every new discovery is the result of expanding the rigid "laws" of the moment. The discovery of the movement of planets, gravity, the circulation of blood, and even infectious diseases all broke the explicable laws of their day, as did Einstein's Relativity Theory. In general, medical "science" accepts as proof or "law" any treatment that is statistically better than placebo, even though most accepted therapies are only a few percentage points better than placebo. No one addresses the wide variation in placebo effectiveness, from 25% up to 90% in some situations![3]

To qualify as a good experiment, each drug or procedure must be evaluated "double-blind" against a placebo. (In a double-blind test, neither the patient nor the researcher knows whether the patient is receiving a drug or a placebo.) I suspect strongly that double-blind evaluation of various placebos would yield some considerably more effective than others! Indeed, one wise man has recently suggested that lactose, the usual placebo, is actually a homeopathic carrier of many antibodies from milk![4]

As Sir William Osler, the Father of American Medicine, said almost a hundred years ago: "Far more important than what the physician does is the patient's belief and the physician's belief in what the physician does."[5] Placebos are thus our most effective therapy!

In general, placebos average 35% effectiveness, but a

number of studies show placebo effectiveness near 50% and a rare one 90%. A drug, to be as effective as a placebo, would thus have to be effective in at least 70% of patients. Most drugs used to treat high blood pressure or depression, however, lead to improvement or control of symptoms 40 to 50% of the time, with 20 to 25% of patients experiencing such severe side effects that they can't take the drug. Side effects are an oxymoronic euphemism for direct physiologic effects of a drug or treatment that are not desired. In other words, no drug is 100% safe, specific, or effective. Even aspirin has in some people such undesirable effects as stomach irritation or bleeding. For simple pain relief, aspirin is much better than the widely promoted acetaminophen. Indeed, although acetaminophen may reduce fever, I think it is primarily a well-advertised placebo in relieving pain.

Actually, I suspect that a placebo, adequately marketed and called a placebo, would be quite effective. And the only risks would be your own fears and doubts!

Conventional medicine has exhausted our belief in the effectiveness of drugs and surgery. Although the conventional approach promises miraculous cures, it often provides only temporary treatment of symptoms and side effects. Fortunately, many alternatives still hold the potential for producing personal miracles. I first became aware of miracles a quarter century ago. Prior to that time, even though miracles occurred regularly, I never noticed them. Actually, they occur in all our lives—almost often enough to cease being miracles. Fortunately, we often don't recognize or acknowledge them, so that the few we actually realize remain numinous enough to grab our attention.

My own introduction to events defying explanation began with an example of synchronicity. At the time, I did not even know the word, created thirty years earlier by Carl Jung. Indeed, science has so rejected this phenomenon that it is not yet in some dictionaries.

Events that seem to be of critical importance in life often occur without a clear cause, as if one pole of a magnet that draws two people together is invisible. Carl Jung called these events synchronicity. Arthur Koestler, in his book, *The Roots of Coincidence,* described this phenomenon even more clearly than did Jung. In the absence of an explicable law of nature, synchronicity is a minor miracle. My personal history thus begins with a brief overview of the synchronistic miracles that have shaped my life for the past three decades.

In the fall of 1976, conscious only of a desire to consider adding to our horse breeding operation, I visited an Appaloosa ranch in Colorado. When Joyce C., wife of the owner, opened the door of their ranch home, I instantly "knew" her, as she did me. The miracle was our instant recognition that we knew one another at a soul level. Joyce and I spent more than an hour discussing synchronicity and parapsychology. After purchasing eight horses, I left forever changed by this brief event.

A week later Joyce sent me *Psychic Discoveries behind the Iron Curtain* and another week later *Breakthrough to Creativity.*[6] These books, after my meeting with Joyce, rekindled an interest in ESP, which I had explored briefly in 1952 when I was asked to write a radio skit for Duke University Campus Radio on the work of Dr. J. B. Rhine. I spent three months observing and interviewing Dr. Rhine, wrote the skit, and then in the fall of 1952 went to medical school. For the next eighteen years, miracle after miracle went by unnoticed.

Such miracles included meeting my future wife, who when I met her was dating my apartment mate. In retrospect, I realize that I was jealous of him from my first meeting with Mary-Charlotte. Perhaps that unacknowledged emotion prevented me from being aware of the unique opportunity to make the most important choice of my life. A few months later, I asked David to stop dating her, because I was sure he would not marry her, and I might! Another month later he agreed on the condition that I not date her for a full month after he ceased. Just one month after we began dating, I asked her to marry me, and considering all the changes, and the fact that she didn't know what had happened, it is probably a miracle that she accepted. In this day of transient relations, it is also miraculous that our marriage has matured into a partnership, the only type of marriage that survives happily.

The miracles of our three children, the first conceived on our first night without contraceptives, were acknowledged only as blessed events. There were also the miracles of two changes of career, the first coming when I chose, after fourteen years of dedication to the goal of being a professor of neurosurgery, to "ruin my career" by leaving the hallowed halls. The second came a year after I met Joyce, when I decided to leave a position as Chief of Neurosciences at one of the ten largest private clinics in America. I had decided to "ruin my career" again by restricting my practice to the management of chronic pain. (These "ruin" statements were made by two close friends.) There was, of course, the miracle of my theorizing in 1965 that electrical stimulation of the spinal cord would control pain. It was so contrary to the laws of science that *The Journal of Neurosurgery* refused to publish my first article on the subject. This led to dorsal column stimulation and transcutaneous electrical nerve stimulation (TENS), both early prototypes of alternative medical devices.

There was the miracle of establishing The Pain Rehabilitation Center, the first use of the concept of "rehabilitating" pain patients which quickly became a popular approach. And then there was the miracle of Dr. Janet Travel, John F. Kennedy's physician, being quoted in *The Wall Street Journal* in January 1972 as mentioning my form of "Western Acupuncture." This mention led to my being invited to visit Dr. Paul Dudley White, Dwight Eisenhower's physician, to discuss my work. In May 1972, I was invited to replace Dr. White on an acupuncture symposium at Stanford University, speaking to an audience of 1,200 professionals.

In April 1972, I had begun planning the first Holistic

Meeting in American Medicine, which was to examine a wide variety of alternative approaches to pain management. I had invited a parapsychologist, Dr. Shafica Karagulla; a spiritual healer; an orgone therapist (another small synchronistic miracle was my wife's gift of *Me and the Orgone*,[7] which opened me to Reichian therapy); two renowned conventional pain experts; an acupuncturist; a chiropractor; and a Christian Scientist practitioner.

The Stanford meeting exposed me to the wide world of alternative miracles, Kirlian photography, subtle energy, spiritual healing, homeopathy, the Edgar Cayce material, and ultimately to autogenic training, biofeedback, Elmer and Alyce Green, and past-life therapy. Bill and Gladys McGarey, holistically and alternatively inclined physicians, whom I met through the Stanford meeting, introduced me to Edgar Cayce's work. In late August 1972, I made my first of two dozen trips to the Association for Research and Enlightenment in Virginia Beach. There I experienced past-life therapy, one of the most effective psychotherapeutic tools available today. (More about this in a later chapter.) I also learned about autogenic training and biofeedback, and I met Dr. Genevieve Haller, a chiropractor who has led me to a variety of alternative ideas, the first being a recommendation that I consult Henry Rucker—my first private experience with an intuitive.

When I entered Henry's office in Chicago, he told me

he'd been waiting ten years for me to show up, as promised by his teacher. He went on, over a three-hour period, to tell me a great deal about my personal life. My work with Henry was the beginning of my involvement with one of the great alternative miracles: intuitive diagnosis. (More about that later.)

Olga Worrall, whom I met at Stanford, introduced me to the field of spiritual healing. This wonderful Sagittarian soul and I had an instant rapport that continued through the rest of her life. At our second meeting a few months later, at a time when she knew nothing about my family, she suddenly said, "Norman, your father is here with a message for you about your sister." The message was clearly a miracle, as Olga did not know that my father was dead or that I had a sister; it was also very emotionally meaningful. Years later Olga suddenly brought me another such message from my father.

A year after meeting Olga, I met, through Dr. Genevieve Haller, the Reverend Bill Brown, an "etheric" surgeon. And in 1976 and 1977 I experienced the most dramatic evidences of spiritual healing: "psychic surgery." These alternative miracles will be discussed later.

Even though I had been cured of an acute sacroiliac problem with a single chiropractic adjustment in 1966, I did not see outside the laws of M.D.s into the miracle of chiropractic (and later osteopathic) treatment until 1979, when Dr. Fred Barge brought our thirteen-year-old daughter's scoliosis under control without the braces and potential surgery of conventional medicine. Although manipulation defies the laws of allopathy (medical doctors), there are, as with many treatments ignored or refused by allopaths, specific facts, quite as real as EKGs or blood sugar, that demonstrate the natural laws of manipulation. Just as the church refused to accept the fact that the earth revolved around the sun instead of the reverse, the refusal of conventional medicine (allopathy, which considers itself the only truth) to accept manipulation is one of the tragedies of modern science. Properly used, manipulation is the treatment of choice in many spinal pain problems.

The miracles of biofeedback became obvious within a few months of my starting to use it, with cures of paraplegic pain, widespread metastatic cancer, and rheumatoid arthritis. Details will be given in later chapters.

Homeopathy remained unacknowledged by me until much later, in 1985, when I learned the Seuterman technique, which is clearly capable of producing many miraculous, scientifically unexplainable cures. Indeed, about 75% of several hundred patients I saw when I visited the Seuterman Clinic claimed homeopathic healing of a variety of illnesses, including multiple sclerosis and rheumatoid arthritis.

Acupuncture, on the other hand, seemed natural and rational to me from the time in 1966 when I began my clinical work with electrical stimulation, or TENS. Rejected by allopathy after the Flexner Report early in this century, acupuncture is perhaps the most likely alternative practice to be grudgingly on the verge of acceptance. It may indeed provide the basis for scientific study of subtle energy, as I shall discuss when we come to GigaTENS, the use of multibillion-hertz electrical frequencies.

Miracles of nutritional approaches are evidenced by much anecdotal evidence, some cases being ones in which cancer or rheumatoid arthritis was reversed. Max Gerson's report of fifty cases of cancer cured with nutrition is only the tip of the iceberg. Once again, I shall in later chapters discuss some of these miracles ignored by conventional medicine.

To a large extent, all the current interest in alternative medicine is a long-delayed acknowledgement by the public that conventional, allopathic medicine has ignored the most important aspect of healing: the untapped miracle of the individual's personal will, intuition, and heart. When will, intuition, and heart are united, even for a few moments, miracles occur. At a deep unconscious level lurks the great suppressed fear inside conventional physicians: Suppose, just suppose, that all those alternatives really work, as well as, or better than, drugs or surgery? And without potentially fatal side effects! Then the power of physicians would evaporate, except for management of acute illness.

It is indeed a miracle gone bad that conventional medicine exists as it does today. Prior to 1900, the likelihood that an M.D. could help most patients was small. In those days, as with Dr. William Osler, physicians primarily provided a good placebo, a boost of morale, hope and belief that something good was being done. Sometimes conventional medicine is no more than pills, prayers, promises, and post-mortems.

Actually, the first major miracle that changed medicine was Alexander Fleming's discovery of penicillin. The frontiers of science were thrown open by this simple mold, which has saved many lives and given us the scientific archetype. Unfortunately, wisdom does not always accompany such discoveries. Just as nuclear energy was a great discovery that in the long run carries the threat of total destruction of life until we learn how to dispose of its waste, antibiotics are now overused and lead to countless allergic reactions. They are used indiscriminately in our food chain, in chickens, cows, and pigs, with unknown long-term outcomes.

The second great scientific miracle, Thorazine, the great root tranquilizer, has produced even broader societal problems. Among other side effects of Thorazine and subsequent new generations of tranquilizers have been two serious complications:

1. The foundation for the problem of homelessness. Patients who are seriously ill emotionally and mentally have been made

placid enough (chemically lobotomized) to be turned out on the streets without rehabilitation.

2. The tranquilization of America. Instead of dealing with stress and anxiety, physicians too often use tranquilizers to suppress the symptoms until patients become addicted and depressed. Indeed, Valium, the next major step in the evolution of tranquilizers, has, in my opinion, harmed many more Americans than marijuana or cocaine. I consider it a hidden plague from which those who care for the Self must remain immune. Once hooked, the journey back to health is formidable.

The list of scientific medical miracles is itself worthy of a large book, but is such a book of any value? Thomas McKeown has emphasized that not more than 8% of the increased longevity Americans enjoy today, compared with 1900, is due to scientific medicine. The other 92% is the result of chlorination of water, proper handling of sewage, pasteurization of milk, and adequate protein![8]

If your auntie were a man, she would be your uncle. In this day when your auntie can "become" a man through the wonders of surgery and hormonal support, what value does such an expensive experiment have for society? Indeed, many of the "miraculous" experiments, such as chemotherapy for most cancers, or transplants of lung, heart, and liver, do nothing for the quality of life and little for the quantity of life. In fact, for the vast majority of chronic illnesses, allopathy may create more harm than good. Among more serious side effects is the slow drugging to death of our elderly.

The root causes of disease are ignored: tobacco, alcohol and drug abuse; obesity; excess fat, salt and sugar; physical inactivity; and the emotional foundations that spawn these habits: fear and its resultant anger, guilt, anxiety, and depression.

If we eliminated the measurable roots of disease, the cost of care could be cut 75%. If we treated the emotional foundations adequately, perhaps 90% of premature illness and death would be eliminated.

A majority of Americans are beginning to feel diseased with the system. They can see that the Emperor (allopathy) has no clothes. Allopathy offers near-miraculous care for most acute illnesses and injuries—with few cures. Given emergency care, the body heals. In the long term, however, allopathy fails to promote and improve health. Instead, it offers mainly side effects and increased chronicity to most illnesses that are untreatable by drugs or surgery. Even conventional psychiatrists today have abandoned their birthright—hypnosis and its related miraculous healings—in favor of tranquilizers and antidepressants, given with too little or no attention to the root cause.

Perhaps it is this feeling of dis-ease with the system that leads Americans to:

1. spend more out-of-pocket money on alternative medicine than on hospitals.

2. make more visits to alternative practitioners than to primary care physicians.[9]

Thus, almost eighty years after Stuart Flexner nearly eradicated alternative medicine, alternative medicine, although ignored and ridiculed by scientific authorities, offers the fastest-growing field of health care.

In one of the few studies of the active uses of folk medicine, Drs. Cheryl Cook and Denise Baisden reported in the *Southern Medical Journal* that 72.9% of 170 individuals surveyed had used at least one folk remedy in the preceding twelve months, with 76% of those from rural areas and 70% of those in urban areas using folk remedies. These particular folk remedies ranged from salt to aloe vera, honey, alcohol, onions, and garlic. Actually, of all these individuals at least 96% reported that they had used folk remedies at some time in their lives, and these folk remedies were generally used to treat symptoms that were considered minor.[10]

Each time a patient recovers during alternative therapy, another miracle is recorded and passed on by word of mouth. The "fact" that Medicine had failed or that some physician had predicted death or worse, without recognizing the healing miracle of the Self, makes such recoveries even more numinous to those who hear of

them. Those who care for themselves and for their friends
and families are not concerned whether the cure is scientific. Whether it works in everyone or just in one, they
appreciate the apparent proof of the pudding. Getting well
is, after all, what it's all about. Forbidden fruit is more
attractive. The more scientific medicine rejects and attacks, the more those who care will be attracted to Expect
a Miracle, See a Miracle, and Accept a Miracle.

The stories of miraculous healings I've seen occur
with a variety of alternative approaches is enough to
produce a whole flock of white crows. Indeed, my experience suggests that all life is a miracle; for life, health, and
illness teach us the remarkable exceptions to the so-
calledlaws of nature. Each of us, holistically viewed—
physically, emotionally, environmentally, and spiritually—is
a miracle far beyond the reach of drugs or surgery. Those
who realize the responsibility of personal care of the Self
will use the miracle of will, mind, and heart to create their
own miracles. Perhaps the fact that you have decided to
read this book will release you to the realization of your
own miraculous future.

FUTURE MIRACLES

Each year creative innovations appear. The most promising, as this is being written, is GigaTENS, about which
you'll read more later.

Ultimately as an adult, anyone eighteen and over must take legal responsibility for virtually every aspect of his or her health. You may consult with any number of experts, talk with unlimited friends or colleagues, read scores of books, but the buck stops here! You can abdicate that responsibility to any number of experts without adequate personal internal dialogue and intuition. In a sense, such reliance on someone else's judgment does not assure any greater success than flipping a coin. Physicians are not God or even near-perfect. They are usually good in diagnosing acute physical and chemical disorders. In serious, life-threatening injuries and diseases, they are often excellent. In such situations, there may be no time for introspection or exploration of alternative approaches.

When the situation becomes chronic, however, you have adequate time to explore all conceivable alternative approaches, from acupuncture to Zen. In some cases, only your intuition can be the final guide.

Obviously, the best solution to health care is the one that optimizes health and prevents disease. Beyond choosing your parents and genes wisely, the others, in order of importance, are:

1. A positive attitude.
2. Avoiding the prime causes of illness (smoking; drug or alcohol abuse; obesity; excess fat, salt, and sugar; the couch potato syndrome).

3. Adequate physical exercise.

4. Good nutrition.

5. Adequate good sleep.

6. Being Care-Full—full of care for yourself to the
   degree adequate to avoid injuries.

The fact that you're reading this book suggests you
are Health Wise. You have already demonstrated that you
care enough to take increasing responsibility for your
health.

As stated in *The Woodrew Update:*

"Science and Miracles! They are both Cosmic
Revelations." So said our cosmic contact, Tauri. If
universal knowledge is available to those who can
tune into it, then the necessary technology will be
available when most needed. A problem to watch
for, however, is that the closer we get to the turn-
of-the-century, the greater the number of prognos-
ticators who surface . . . those who predict. Every
town has its channelers who'll tell you what you
want to hear, from whom you'll meet . . . to what
you'll eat. You may find them fun, but know them
for who they are.

   "Inventing is a form of channeling," wrote
Joseph Whitfield in *The Treasure of El Dorado.* Tauri
agreed. Many scientists are recipients of cosmic

information through a technique which can only be described as mental imagery projection. An actual picture is projected through the subconscious mind. It produces a glimmer or vibration within the consciousness. "Then," said Whitfield, "The conscious mind translates the projection into a picture image in much the same way a TV set does." Greta does it, and calls it her "destiny screen." It enables her to use knowledge outside of linear time that is unavailable to her otherwise. Many of you have observed Greta during this process.

Through the years, COSMIC REVELATION has been connected to many of science's greatest bursts of achievement. Sir Isaac Newton invented calculus and developed his theory of gravity at the age of 23, during the plague-ridden years of 1665 and 1666. Columbia University historian Lynn Thorndyke compared Newton's method of discovery to "that of a medium coming out of a trance." Lord John Maynard Keynes, speaking at the Tercentenary of Newton in 1947 said, "His deepest instincts were occult, esoteric, semantic . . . with a profound shrinking from the world." It sounds like the mental imagery projection method.

Science 1984 called Dr. Albert Einstein the greatest scientist of the 20th century. They wrote, "The Einstein who celebrated his 26th birthday on

March 14, 1905, was nobody's candidate for distinction. A high school dropout, he had squeaked through college with a B average, skipping classes and cramming for final examinations with a friend's lecture notes. Five years passed since his graduation from the Polytechnic Academy in Zurich, and still no university would employ him. He worked in the Swiss patent office in Bern. Yet, before the year 1905 was out, Einstein had written six epochal papers that transformed the scientific landscape. Two of them created a new branch of physics: relativity. A third helped create quantum physics. The other three altered the course of atomic theory and statistical mechanics. Not since Isaac Newton in 1665–66 had science witnessed such a burst of creativity."

Then there was Thomas Edison, holder of over 1000 patents, including the electric bulb, phonograph, and motion-picture projector. *Search* magazine wrote that "much of what he put down on paper originated from a higher source, and that he was simply a vehicle or channel through which this information could flow freely." Experts who have examined his original papers feel that much of his work resembles automatic writing. Add in the achievements of Nicola Tesla and Guglielmo Marconi . . . prize-winning physicists who openly acknowledged a cosmic assist in their work and you make a solid case for Science and Miracles being cosmic revelations. You can also understand the process that allows necessary technology to be available when most needed.

What makes a miracle a miracle? Perhaps the answer is our ignorance of what occurs. If we knew how Nature really works, we wouldn't call such phenomena "miracles" at all. In fact the only real miracle is life! Authentic mystics will tell you that there really is nothing metaphysical in the world. Quoting Kyriacos Markides, author of *Fire in the Heart,* "It is the limitation of our awareness that would classify certain phenomena or abilities as metaphysical. Our awareness about what Nature is all about is grossly limited. Whatever is outside these limitations we tend to call metaphysical and then define as something beyond the scope of science and reason."

In other words, we consider "natural" and "real" only what is accessible to our basic and ordinary senses: to sight, touch, taste, hearing and smell. But we are not simply the product of five gross senses! We can surely agree that we are capable of going beyond them, and that we can extend our awareness, our senses, our capabilities. We can raise our consciousness and our lower vibrations. We recognize that mind can move matter. We know that we are capable of evolving into control of our health and welfare. Mystical? Magical? Not at all . . . not at all.[11]

NOTES

1. D.M. Eisenberg, et al., "Unconventional Medicine in the United States: Prevalence, Costs, and Patterns of Use," *New England Journal of Medicine* (January 28, 1994) 4: 246–256).

2. Bernard S. Cayne, ed., *The New Lexicon Webster's Dictionary of the English Language* (New York: Lexicon, 1987).

3. Herb Benson, "Angina Pectoris and the Placebo Effect," *New England Journal of Medicine* 300 (June 21, 1979): 1424–29.

4. Paul Weighner, personal conversation with author.

5. Sir William Osler, *Aequanimitas*, 3rd ed. (Philadelphia: Blakiston, 1943).

6. Sheila Ostranter, *Psychic Discoveries behind the Iron Curtain* (Englewood Cliffs, NJ: Prentice Hall, 1970); Shafica Karagulla, *Breakthrough to Creativity* (Los Angeles: De Vorss, 1967).

7. Orson Bean, *Me and the Orgone* (New York: St. Martin's, 1971).

8. Thomas McKeown, *The Role of Medicine, Mirage or Nemesis* (London: Nuffield Provincial Hospitals Trust, 1976).

9. Eisenberg, et al., "Unconventional Medicine in the United States: Prevalence, Costs, and Patterns of Use."

10. Drs. Cheryl Cook and Denise Baisden reported in the *Southern Medical Journal* 79 (September 1986): 1098–1101.

11. *The Woodrew Update* 14 (Nov/Dec 1994) 2:6. Reprinted by permission of the publisher.

Chapter 2

Intuitive Diagnosis

All our moments add together
Like the digits in a sum,
And the answer tells us plainly
Whether life or death shall come.
—Anonymous

> There is a limit beyond which
> forbearance ceases to be a virtue.
> —Aurobindo

Human affection is obviously unreliable
because it is so much based upon
selfishness and desire.
—Aurobindo

Accurate intuition, by its very nature, challenges the laws of nature as defined today by science. There simply is no law acceptable to conventional scientists that allows for the possibility of knowing something without having facts behind that knowledge. Quantum physicists are the exception; like Rupert Sheldrake and David Bohm, they have little difficulty with the possibility of tuning into a morphogenic field or to the collective unconscious intuited so brilliantly by Carl Jung.

The terms "morphogenic field" and "collective unconscious" suggest the existence of a subtle electromagnetic framework or pervasive background of information. Just as television and radio signals go through us without our conscious awareness, we are surrounded by the "signals" of information, especially of great emotional common experiences. These signals, ignored by the conscious mind, are available to the intuitive mind. If your mind functions as a super-receiver, it is able to tune in to this information.

In reality, every great invention, every scientific breakthrough, every masterpiece of art or music is the result of intuition. Dr. J.B. Rhine at Duke University proved that some individuals can know intuitively which card is being drawn by another person—not 100% of the time but at a rate that is significantly greater than chance.

A hundred years before Rhine, two of the fathers of hypnosis, John Elliotson and James Esdaile, demonstrated that some individuals enjoyed an inherent clairvoyance great enough to make medical diagnoses without medical training. Elliotson in particular demonstrated repeatedly that individuals placed in a mesmeric trance could make accurate diagnoses.[1] Even in their day, however, the Establishment rejected the concept without bothering to study it adequately.

Then, in the first half of this century, Edgar Cayce provided a remarkable opportunity for proof of intuitive diagnosis. In almost 15,000 readings given while he was in trance, Cayce, a photographer with no medical training, gave diagnosis after diagnosis, treatment after treatment, often with uncanny success. Today scores of books delve into the Cayce material, and a few hundred physicians and chiropractors use various remedies that Cayce recommended.

One of the most intriguing Cayce remedies was his recommendation of castor oil packs on the abdomen to relieve a variety of conditions, including lymph in need of cleansing. In recent years, scientific studies have confirmed that castor oil packs enhance some aspects of the immune lymphocyte system. A truly miraculous prescription by Cayce.

I have used castor oil packs successfully to heal wounds on horses that had been recommended for euthanasia because veterinarians thought they were hopeless. And castor oil packs on a swollen knee work faster to reduce the swelling than does a shot of cortisone. Much safer, too! A castor oil pack on the abdomen in a case of intestinal flu brings relief of pain and bloating faster than does any known drug.

Cayce's legacy, standing alone, provides more examples of miracles than the modern pharmacy. But it is in the field of intuitive diagnosis that miracles abound, not just with Cayce but with several contemporary intuitives.

Actually, as Dr. Irvine Page, the great Cleveland Clinic internist, wrote wisely almost two decades ago, intuition is the key to diagnosis by the most competent physicians.[2] How else can one choose between thousands of potential diagnoses?

In fact, I made my first obviously intuitive diagnosis when I was a junior medical student. One weekend I diagnosed an extremely rare condition, sarcoidosis of the pituitary gland. This uncommon granulomatous disease, appearing under the microscope much like tuberculosis but without an infectious agent, had not been diagnosed at Duke before this time. The attending physician exclaimed that I couldn't make such a diagnosis because I was too young. But I did. He and I subsequently wrote a definitive paper on the subject, including a report on four such cases!

It can be argued, of course, that I at least had a significant amount of education and the advantage of a case history and a personal physical examination of the patient. Never mind that several more experienced physicians had failed to make the diagnosis. But in the case of Henry Rucker, how could he, with no medical training and only two years of college, diagnose several hundred patients with better than 70% accuracy just from seeing a photograph?

Henry first visited me in January 1973. One among other diagnoses he performed was to correctly discern the cause of paralysis in three patients paralyzed from chest down by three different causes: infection, gunshot, and auto accident. And in one patient whose white blood count of more than 40,000 had led us to search for leukemia, Henry correctly diagnosed liver dysfunction from a recent anesthetic. A miracle?

In addition to several hundred accurate diagnoses, Henry is a superb counselor and healer. The most remarkable healing I saw Henry perform was of a spreading skull fracture in a young child. Surgery was being contemplated, but Henry laid hands on the child and subsequently worked with a photograph to produce a healing impossible with drugs.

In the case of a sixteen-year-old boy deeply involved with drugs and a failure in several drug programs, Henry spent only an hour with him. Afterwards the young man said to his parents, "Why didn't anyone ever talk to me like that before?" The patient remained free of drugs and went on to become motivated and successful. If he had continued in conventional programs, I expect that he would still be an addict today.

After I had tested Henry initially, I received a grant of $50,000 from a Fortune 500 company to study intuitive diagnosis, with the requirement that I not divulge the name of the company! In retrospect, the very idea of such a grant seems miraculous.

As part of my study in 1973, I investigated seventy-five intuitives. All of them proved to be about 50% accurate; the possibility of being right by chance is only 5 to 10%. Although such findings are highly significant statistically, they are of little clinical use. Henry's 70% success rate is almost as good as that of a competent physician who has the advantages of knowing the patient's history and having given a physical examination. These two advantages give physicians an 80% chance of being accurate before they test further. Five other non-medically trained intuitives whom I studied that year proved to be from 70 to 75% accurate in their diagnoses–by the laws of nature, these are miracles.

Then, in January 1974, I became acquainted with Dr. Robert Leichtman, an internist, whose accuracy on physical diagnosis was 80% and in psychological diagnoses 96%–just by hearing the patient's name and birth date, address, or telephone number! Bob's accuracy is truly miraculous. Of course, when he misses, he misses–just as do physicians 20% of the time initially, and even sometimes after thousands of dollars' worth of sophisticated tests. I have consulted Bob on hundreds of cases in which I had reached an impasse in diagnosis. One outstanding example was of a man with sacroiliac pain and no tenderness above the fourth lumbar vertebra. Bob said to look at L2. When I placed a needle on the L2 facet, under fluoroscopy, the patient yelled, "That's it," and responded well to my treatment.

In another case, when a young woman entered my office, I saw in the energy around her a chaotic storm–something I have grown to recognize as typical of psychosis. (I've always seen energy around people. It looks like heat waves with movement and sometimes color.) I sent the woman to my waiting room and phoned Bob. I gave the patient's name and told him she was in my waiting room. "Oh, yes," he said, "she's a simple paranoid schizophrenic." She had not been diagnosed by a cardiologist in Detroit, who sent her to see me for pain control. I had her evaluated by a psychiatrist, who confirmed the diagnosis. In general, even to this date, I have seen few miracle cures of schizophrenia, and the chaotic nature of such patients' energy makes it difficult for me to be in their presence. But such a diagnosis over the phone? That's a miracle.

After working with Bob for ten years, I met Caroline Myss, with whom I've now worked closely for the past ten years. In physical or psychological diagnoses, Caroline is accurate 93% of the time. To make her diagnoses, Caroline needs only the patient's name and age; she's better at making a diagnosis by phone than she is in person, where her emotional concern for the patient may interfere. Interestingly, Caroline can perform a maximum of eight diagnoses in a given day. It's as if her computer gets overloaded after eight successes.

Caroline also has given me hundreds of correct diagnoses, each a miracle in the sense of defying the known laws of nature. A few examples may illustrate the benefits and pitfalls of using intuitive diagnosis.

A forty-year-old woman consulted me to obtain possible alternative ways to control severe non-menstrual vaginal bleeding. Her gynecologist had recommended hysterectomy for fibroid tumors. With the patient's permission, I phoned Caroline while the patient sat in my office. Caroline said, "Did she tell you about her two abortions?" The patient had not, and when confronted gently with the unfinished business of her two abortions, she refused to deal with the issue and left immediately.

Or take the case of Jack, a fifty-year-old contractor who had rammed into a car that sat across an interstate highway as Jack came over a hilltop. The driver of the car had earlier hit five cows, and a coroner determined that the driver was dead before Jack's truck hit the car. Despite knowing this, Jack went into a deep depression. Several physicians had failed to help either Jack's spinal pain or his depression, and everything I tried also failed. I finally phoned Caroline, who said, "If he doesn't come out of his depression within a year, he'll have cancer of the intestine." At that time, Jack had no intestinal symptoms, and I did not share with him this bit of Caroline's conversation. She made some suggestions about his need to deal with poor self-esteem. Nothing worked, and three months later Jack was operated on for cancer of the colon. Several months later, in February, Jack was still in the pits. When I consulted Caroline again, she said, "If he doesn't come out of depression, he'll be dead in August." This time I decided to try verbal shock therapy and told him her prediction. I also shared with him my notes of the previous year. Still nothing worked, including several different antidepressants. Jack died August 31 of the *following* year. (I had forgotten to ask Caroline which August.)

More positive is the case of the wealthy European woman with severe throat numbness from polyneuropathy. She presented a medically untreatable problem: there has simply been no medical "cure" for diabetic neuropathy. Caroline suggested that this was a karmic illness from a past life in which this woman had died from a blunt blow to the throat. Without telling the patient this diagnosis, I simply suggested that Caroline recommended past-life therapy. I induced a light trance in the patient and asked her to return to the life in which she had unfinished business related to her throat. She gave a story of being a Polynesian teenager kidnapped by pirates. While she was imprisoned beneath deck, the pirate's ship was attacked and began to sink; a large beam floated over and pinned her throat against the wall, asphyxiating her.

Following the session, my patient decided she needed to divorce her husband, whom she suspected of sexually abusing her sons. Although Caroline had not mentioned the connection to the throat chakra or energy center, this area of the body is clearly associated with expression of will. Once my patient expressed her will, she recovered sensation in her throat! Two miracles for the price of one: Caroline's diagnosis and the healing of polyneuropathy.

Such is the heady stuff of intuitive diagnosis. Much more commonly, however, I have seen individuals who acknowledge the validity of Caroline's diagnosis or re-marks about root cause nevertheless refuse, or be unable, to make the changes necessary to accomplish healing. Actually, I suspect this same block is responsible for the

abominably low rate of cure with conventional psychoanalysis. Patients wallow in their psychic manure for many
years and refuse to make the changes necessary to effect
cure.

Problems are generally simple. Patients feel abandoned or abused. Their fear from such experiences leads
them to react with anger, guilt, anxiety, and/or depression.
They are unable or unwilling to forgive the abuser, often
bury primary feelings, and go on suffering. Whether they
spend days, months, or years in therapy, the only solutions
are:

1. Assertion–The Fight Response. Abused people
   have a right to fight back, to tell the abuser how
   much they have been hurt, and to demand an
   apology or retribution. Of course, the abuser
   may refuse, may become angry, or may already
   be deceased.

2. Flight–Divorce with Joy. If the abusive relationship is ongoing, especially if there is physical
   abuse, the only reasonable solution is separa-
   tion from the abuser.

3. Go with the Flow–Go for Sainthood. Accept
   and forgive. Ultimately, those things that cannot be changed must be accepted. And holding
   a grudge harms only the person already
   abused. Unfortunately, many persons feel they
   have a right to be upset. And indeed they do,

but for what good? Ultimately, healing begins with forgiveness—of others and of self. Forgiveness cán produce miracles, as you'll read later. Telling a hurt person this truism, however, is virtually useless. The patient must have a deep emotional feeling of forgiveness and reach into the Soul for strength to heal.

About 1990, I decided that intuitive diagnosis by Caroline or me, or even medical/psychological diagnosis, was of little value unless the patient had the personal intuitive, "Aha!"

So Caroline and I set about teaching patients to reach their own intuitive knowing of cause and of solution. The results have been even more miraculous than those obtained previously with Caroline or other talented intuitives. At least 74% of chronically depressed patients so instructed have achieved long-term relief of their long-standing depression, which had previously failed to respond to drugs. Such statistics are themselves miraculous, for they are better than the results of any antidepressant drugs, and they have no risky side effects. Details of this alternative program will be provided in a later chapter. Nevertheless, intuitive diagnosis, whether done by you or by a talented intuitive person, provides many possibilities for experiencing miracles—events that exceed the laws of nature.

Caroline Myss and I began teaching a course called "The Science of Intuition" in 1991. We regularly conduct a ten-day, two-part, course that is designed to provide a foundation for the flow of natural creativity and intuition. Some of our students have become medically intuitive; others have blossomed in their careers. The principles outlined in my earlier book, *The Self-Healing Workbook*, offer you a basic home study course for developing your own intuition. Caroline's forthcoming book, *The Anatomy of Power*, and our joint book to follow, *Sacred Contracts*, will add further information to expand your personal growth. Meanwhile, if you want to study with us, contact Self-Health Systems, 5607 South 222nd Road, Fair Grove, MO 65648.

Ultimately, everyone can experience miracles if they open themselves to the abundant opportunity to observe synchronicity. The greatest block to miracles is unfinished emotional anguish—fears, anger, guilt, anxiety and/or depression. Once you banish these negative responses, the miracle of life itself is constantly inspiring.

NOTES

1. James Esdaile, *Natural and Mesmeric Clairvoyance* (London: H. Balliere, 1852).

2. Irvine H. Page, "Science, Intuition and Medical Practice," *Post-Graduate Medicine* 64 (November 1978) 217–221.

Chapter 3

Self-Regulation, Biofeedback, and Biogenics

These things and more you shall do.
–Jesus of Nazareth, John 14:12

> Any moment of hating,
> Any moment of lying,
> Any moment of resentment,
> Is a moment of dying.
> –Anonymous

Any moment of loving,
Any moment of giving,
Any moment of thankfulness,
Is a moment of living.
–Anonymous

The practice of feeding back to the student visual or audible information to assist learning has been used for centuries. In the late 1960s, Dr. Elmer Green and his wife, Alyce, took this concept a major step forward, feeding back physiologic activity to patients to show them their internal reactions. They concentrated on skin temperature, which is a reflection of blood flow and an indication of reaction to stress. In a stressful state, the fight-or-flight response leads to constriction of the blood vessels in the extremities (hand, foot, arm, leg) and subsequent coolness. In patients suffering migraine headaches, the blood vessels in the hands usually constrict and those at the base of the brain usually dilate. A normal reflex can be activated when the hands are warmed internally, a process leading to narrowing of the blood vessels at the base of the brain to their normal size and thus bringing the headache under control. Warming the hands by placing them in warm water fails to work, because the neural reflex requires the switch to take place in the sympathetic nervous system, presumably involving at least the ganglia controlling blood flow to the arms and head.

Long before biofeedback training, Edgar Cayce called the sympathetic system the imaginative nervous system, for he realized that it is indeed responsive to images. Actually, of course, we think and feel only in images. Words are substitutes for images.

Anxiety triggers our stored memories of fear and prepares us for fight or flight. Blood is shifted to the muscles so that they can work more efficiently. Alyce and Elmer used the principle of information feedback to teach patients temperature/blood flow control. If you train your nervous system by saying repetitively, "My hands are warm," and at the same time imagine the sun beaming pleasantly down upon your hands, then your hands will become warm. Normal skin temperature in a room warmed to only seventy or seventy-two degrees is eighty-four to ninety degrees Fahrenheit.

With practice, using only a simple thermometer taped to the index finger, with the outer surface of the thermometer's bulb exposed to air, people can learn to warm their hands to ninety-six or even ninety-eight degrees. Daily practice with words, images, and thermometer feedback, for fifteen minutes two to four times a day leads to control within a week or two. Continued practice for three to six months leads to marked reduction in frequency and severity of migraine headaches in 80% of patients.

It appears that most of those who fail to control their migraines in this way do so because they do not practice or because they doubt their ability. Those who continue to use temperature feedback still have control of their migraines more than five years later. This simple, effective alternative to drug therapy for migraine is by far the safest and most successful treatment known for migraine. Considering the failure of conventional physicians and the insurance industry to recommend or pay for biofeedback training, biofeedback remains one of the alternative miracles.

The Greens also demonstrated that people who learn to warm their toes to ninety-six degrees bring high blood pressure under control 80% of the time! Dr. Green says those who learn to warm their toes *always* improve their blood pressure. Despite twenty years of corroborative research, temperature biofeedback remains largely rejected by the medical profession and medical insurance companies. To these mentally unimaginative beings, such cures are miracles, for they transgress the rules of their drug/surgery world!

When I heard Dr. Green speak on the benefits of temperature biofeedback in January 1993, I phoned and asked him whether it could be used to control back pain. He had not used biofeedback for that problem but suggested I try it. So I purchased EEG (electroencephalogram or brain wave), EMG (electromyogram or muscle tension), and temperature feedback devices and began using them with autogenic training, which I had started using in the fall of 1972.

Autogenic training was begun in the early 1900s by J.H. Schultz, a German psychiatrist, who wished to make his patients less dependent upon him. He found that patients who were in hypnotic trances reported feeling:

- heavy arms, hands, legs, and feet
- warm arms, hands, legs, and feet
- calm regularity of the heartbeat
- complete freedom in breathing, as if the breathing were automatic

- warmth in the abdomen
- coolness of the forehead.

When patients were instructed to repeat the phrases:

My arms and legs are heavy and warm.

My heartbeat is calm and regular.

My breathing is free and easy.

My abdomen is warm.

My forehead is cool.

for 10 to 15 minutes twice a day over a period of six months, 80% of patients with a wide variety of psychosomatic or stress illnesses improved markedly: miracles, from the allopathic point of view.

By 1969, seven books had been published on autogenic training, and more than 2,600 scientific articles were in press investigating various effects of autogenic training in a wide variety of illnesses as well as in enhancing results in students, business people, and athletes. Autogenic training was widely used in Europe and Japan to train Olympic athletes.

Despite this scientific background and the support of research on the benefits of autogenic training and biofeedback, conventional medicine continues to ignore the most successful single alternative technique known to date!

One of my cases in which I used biofeedback in a patient taught me something new. Early in 1973 Lawrence, a fifty-year-old man, came to me with severe paraplegic pain syndrome and pain in his pelvis when he sat up, despite the fact that his spinal cord was transected at the second thoracic spinal level. For seven years he had been unable to sit up for more than fifteen minutes at a time.

Two days after beginning biofeedback, Lawrence reported that he could sit comfortably for four hours after each fifteen minute biofeedback session.

"How did you do it?" I asked.

He could say only, "It's as if I threw a switch in my brain."

I set out to learn how to throw the switch. In order to understand the root of this miracle of pain control, over the next year I read three hundred books in the field of self-regulation. Please understand that conventional drugs and surgery, even cutting out an inch of spinal cord, cannot control paraplegic pain!

As I read, I began to synthesize a method by which we can control our bodies and minds. Optimal personal control involves the following steps:

Focus of Attention

Center upon NOW, letting go of concerns about past, present, or future.

Belief in Self

This means belief that you can do it. Biofeedback is

particularly helpful here, for the simple machines show you that if you think and image properly, the body responds properly.

Temperature biofeedback is particularly useful in all forms of pain control, for temperature and pain sensations travel in the spinal cord in exactly the same pathways. Control of temperature thus quickly leads to control of pain.

A Positive Attitude

Negativity produces stress. There are only two attitudes–positive or negative. Negative attitudes are the result of fear of loss of life, health, love, or existential issues. Fear leads to the fight-or-flight response. Positive attitudes of joy and love are nurturing. Everyone knows the power of positive thinking; practice living it.

The Relaxation Response

Dr. Herb Benson demonstrated that deep relaxation, practiced twenty minutes twice a day leads to a 50%, twenty-four hour reduction in adrenalin, the hormone that stress releases, and 50% reduction in the amount of insulin required.[1] Relaxation is the natural result of focus of attention on any thought or image that is not stressful. Relaxation reduces muscle tension to a minimum.

Remember that all pain is either partly or totally the result of muscle tension.

Conscious Control of Sensation

Physical sensations can be changed by a variety of mental techniques. Of course, one has first to learn to feel. Many people have habitually blocked feelings because of being told such things as, "Big boys don't cry." They believe that acknowledging their feelings is not manly, or even womanly, since women as well as men learn to ignore feelings (emotional/physical sensations resulting from mental attitudes). Most of us thus learn to ignore almost all physical sensations or feelings. Once you learn to tune in and accept physical feelings, you learn that:

- Feelings change constantly in every part of the body.
- There are always some sensations in each part of the body.
- You can focus on feeling or not feeling any part of the body.
- You can change from one feeling to another.
- You can, therefore, create feelings, or sensations.
- You can choose what you feel and when you feel it.

If you want to control your mind and body in this way, you may try the nine major techniques I have selected to assist the process of conscious control of sensations:

1. *Talk to the body.* The foundation of this concept is autogenic training. If you speak the words repetitively long enough, the body will respond.

2. *Visualize the desired result.* If you want your hands to be warm, image a pleasantly warm sunbeam on that part of the body, or think of holding them in front of a cozy fireplace or heater.

3. *Feel the pulse.* Every cell pulsates every time your heart beats. Only when there is tension in a given part does blood flow reduce enough to block feelings. Wilhelm Reich called this "armoring," since it is usually caused by local muscle tension, which constricts blood flow, just as armor does.

4. *Love it.* Most people with any dysfunction dislike the part of the body that is ill. You can't afford to hate any part of your body. Rejection of a part of the body causes muscle tension and vasoconstriction. Loving a part of the body creates a warm, fuzzy, pleasant, healthy feeling.

5. *Tense and relax.* Edmund Jacobson, an American physician, published his great book, *Progressive Relaxation,* in 1929.[2] He demonstrated that 80% of psychosomatic or stress illnesses could be markedly improved just by practicing progres-

sive relaxation thirty minutes a day. His technique was slow and consistent, starting with a
small group of muscles and systematically
contracting and relaxing muscle groups through
the entire body.

You can demonstrate easily to yourself
the change in feeling caused by releasing tension if you first notice the sensations in your
right hand and arm and then make a tight fist.
Note the feelings of tension and the way they
spread to the jaws and entire body. Take a deep
breath and let go of the tension in your right
hand. Experience the change in feelings/sensa-
tions in your right hand and arm.

6. *Collect and release tension.* Breathe in and imag-
    ine collecting tension from your feet, then
    breathe out, releasing the tension. Do this
    systematically through each part of the body.
    This is one of the quickest methods for letting
    go of tension and/or any undesired sensation.
    The technique was used by Native Americans
    as preparation for meditation.

7. *Breathe through the skin.* This East Indian tech-
    nique is one of the most effective for pain
    control. Imagine air is being breathed in and
    out through any one part of the body. After
    fifteen to twenty minutes focused on one area,
    that area becomes quite numb or anesthetized.

8. *Visualize circulating electrical energy.* Every activity within the body or mind is electrical. Imagine circulating this energy from your heels up your entire back to the top of your head as you breathe in, and circulating the electrical energy down over the front of your body as you breathe out. You will notice some areas where the feeling of flow is absent. Concentrate on these areas over and over to open the circuits of sensation.

9. *Expand the electromagnetic field.* Electricity creates magnetism. Imagine a one-inch halo of living electromagnetic energy around your feet. Slowly allow this capsule of electromagnetic energy to flow around your legs, buttocks, pelvis, abdomen, chest, shoulders, arms, hands, neck, and head. Then repeat, expanding your electromagnetic halo to twelve inches, around the entire body. It is impossible to feel pain when this state is entered. You feel as if your mind is alert and awake; the body is numb or floating.

Practicing one or more of these nine techniques fifteen minutes twice a day not only gives deep relaxation but increases your balance/harmony of feeling/sensation and of function. When you finish the session, however, any fear, anger, guilt, anxiety, or sadness will re-create

tension and dysfunction. Thus the next step is crucial to
maintaining health.

Conscious Control of Emotion/Attitudes

As I've said before, it is natural to be upset if you are
abused. If you are seriously threatened, anger awakens the
fight-or-flight response. Anger then serves to protect you,
if you deal with it appropriately. If you simply allow anger
to fester, then you are at great risk of eventual physical
illness. Even conventional medicine is coming to recognize this fact.

> Psychological stress was associated in a dose-
> response manner with an increased risk of acute
> infectious respiratory illness, and this risk was
> attributable to increased rates of infection rather
> than to an increased frequency of symptoms after
> infection.[3]

All negative feelings consist of anger, guilt, anxiety,
depression, or related emotions. One needs to practice
bringing up negative emotions–unfinished business–to
the surface of consciousness, then feeling the tension and
letting go of it. Eventually through a variety of Gestalt-like
symbolic exercises, we can train our bodies and minds to
let go of undesired feelings or emotions, to forgive those
who have wronged us, to accept what cannot be changed,
and to be at peace. There are literally dozens of guided or

active imagination exercises that assist the process of emotional attitudinal healing. As noted in an earlier chapter, the goal is to:

Change the things you can,

Divorce the things you cannot, and

Be at peace with everything.

Forgiveness is often the trigger for miracles. Resentment and judgmentalism prevent miracles.

The process of forgiveness is simple but not easy. Some individuals learn it within a few days; others require months of practice. In a later chapter on depression, I will describe an insight meditation chamber that seems to speed up the process of emotional resolution and balance.

Programming Goals

Once you have learned control of feelings and emotions, not burying or denying but playing with them, then you can change other physiological tensions much more quickly. You can do this by setting a goal, stated as though already attained, for instance, "My blood pressure is 120/80."

It is important to create a simple, short, positive goal, worded not to state what you want to get rid of but what you want to create.

Create a positive, emotionally meaningful goal, preferably in six words (the maximum is twelve). Create an image to go with it. Many of my patients have created miracles with this technique.

Spiritual Attunement

The goal of each human is ultimately to be in tune with the Soul, the higher or inner Self, the Ideal. This ideal acknowledges at all levels that the only great commandment is the Golden Rule. No other goal is as soul-satisfying.

Many varieties of guided or active imagination can be used to create experiences of being transcendent of body and mind and at one with the Soul or God.

I call these techniques Biogenics, and if I were restricted to only one mode of healing, it would be the integrated approach, for in dealing with the most difficult patients suffering a wide variety of chronic pains, I have seen many miracles accomplished with it. In more than 9,000 patients suffering from chronic pain of various types, 70% experience gratifying relief on a long-term basis. Another 15% of patients who achieved good relief initially were unable to muster the will to continue the regular practice necessary to maintain improvement.

A few case reports, cited below, show the potential for miracle cures with this sort of self-regulation.

A fifty-year-old Black woman I'll call A.Z. arrived on April 30, 1974, with generalized back pain and massively widespread metastatic cancer of the breast. Her oncologist had told her family she had, at best, three months to live;

I was not certain she'd last three weeks! She was so weak she could not walk; she vomited most of her food. Her body was further weakened by extensive radiation therapy and chemotherapy, which had failed to slow her cancer.

She was annoyed at the idea of retraining the nervous system. She complained, "I didn't come here to be brainwashed; I came to get rid of my pain." I replied, "If you would just listen, I'll teach you how to control your pain."

On the seventeenth day of treatment, I performed with A.Z. a guided exercise on forgiveness. She had been brought into the room on a stretcher, but after the experience she arose and walked out of the room free of pain. It was like a scene from Lourdes; half the people in the room were in tears.

Three months later A.Z.'s cancer was totally gone, never to return. She made a silk screen seriograph with a sketch of a pop bottle labeled "Dr. Shealy," and the slogan, "Autogenics–The Pause That Refreshes." This remarkable healing proved to me that Miracles Do Happen. Forgiveness was the trigger.

Not until a year and a half later did I learn just what had happened to her. In December 1975, I was in California to deliver a lecture and A.Z. picked me up at the airport. She was radiantly happy and healthy. As we were riding down a freeway she said,

> During that exercise, I suddenly realized how
> much I hated my family. I decided not to let the

bastards kill me! When I got home, I said to my husband, "I'm going to get well!" He replied, "But A.Z., you've got cancer, you're going to die!" I got well, and four months later he committed suicide.

In late 1976, A.Z.'s pet dog died and she became very depressed. Her back pain returned and she came back to see me. I could find no evidence of cancer. When I was working with her on this occasion she said, "I realize now that I cannot afford the luxury of depression." What a wise observation! No one can afford the luxury of depression— or any other unresolved negative emotion. Her miracle cure began with a simple decision of will.

Another case of mine was cured of rheumatoid arthritis by means of Biogenics. In July 1994, B.Y., a woman of about fifty years of age, came up to me at a lecture I was giving in Boston. She asked if I remembered her from ten years previously when she came to my clinic suffering from rheumatoid arthritis and a stomach irritated by drugs. She reported having no symptoms of rheumatoid arthritis and attributed her entire cure to Biogenics, even though she could not recall a dramatic emotional insight that contributed to her relief. Basically, she was certain that overall her cure came about as a result of her relief of general stress overload, handled with Biogenics. There are, incidentally, no miracle cures of rheumatoid arthritis with drugs, which sometimes control symptoms but are generally accompanied by a high price in complications.

In November 1975, C.X., a sixty-year-old Franco-

American woman, came to me with active rheumatoid arthritis and many hot, swollen joints, despite five years of treatments with cortisone and gold shots. On the seventh day of our twelve-day training program, she said, "Dr. Shealy, I don't have rheumatoid arthritis any more."

"How do you know, C.X.?" I replied.

"When you've had rheumatoid arthritis five years and it goes away, you know!" The implication of her remark was, "Of course I know, stupid." She was right. Her joints were no longer swollen, hot, or red.

On the twelfth day, as I was dictating a final summary, she said,

> I want to tell you about my rheumatoid arthritis. I've been married twenty-five years. My husband has been unfaithful since we were married. I learned about it when our third son was born but I decided to stick out the marriage until our sons were grown. When our third son was eighteen, he was drafted and sent to Vietnam with his two brothers. I couldn't divorce their father while they were in Vietnam. I developed rheumatoid arthritis.
>
> When they came home safely from Vietnam, I couldn't divorce their father because I was an invalid; who would take care of me? And I kept saying to myself, if it weren't for that blankety-blank S.O.B., I wouldn't have rheumatoid arthritis. What I realized here is that my husband did not create my rheumatoid arthritis; I did, through my

attitude towards him. I've decided I don't want to divorce my husband. I love him, and I think he loves me. I don't like his affairs, but they are his problem, not mine.

Forgiveness created her miracle.

I saw C.X. five years later while I was lecturing near her home and she was still totally free of rheumatoid arthritis.

In 1981, a nineteen-year-old woman came to me with phantom leg pain, which was poorly managed by codeine. Phantom limb pain is similar to paraplegic pain—impossible to control with drugs or surgery. This bright young woman learned total control of her pain and came off codeine within four days. She could then control her pain with just fifteen minutes of Biogenics practice each morning.

Of all the self-care techniques, none is superior to Biogenics. There are no side effects; it is totally safe; and it can work in any illness. All it requires is belief and practice—the foundations for creating your own miracles. And for spiritual healing!

NOTES

1. Herbert Benson, *The Relaxation Response* (New York: Avon, 1975).

2. Edmund Jacobson, *Progressive Relaxation* (Chicago: University of Chicago Press, 1929).

3. Sheldon Cohen, David A.J. Tyrrell, and Andrew P. Smith, "Psychological Stress and Susceptibility to the Common Cold," *New England Journal of Medicine* 325 (August 1991): 606–612.

Chapter 4

Spiritual Healing

Another little touch of healing
never hurt anyone. . . .
Diabetes was never cured
with a single shot of insulin.
—Olga Worrall

A divine life and a divine body
is the formula of the ideal.
—Aurobindo

Prayer is the medium of miracles . . .
Through prayer love is received,
and through miracles love is expressed.
—*A Course in Miracles*

Not to kill the emotion, but to turn it
in toward the Divine is the right way.
—Aurobindo

The laying on of hands and the offering of prayers for
healing are probably as old as humanity. People from

ancient priests and kings to modern healers like Olga
Worrall have reported quiet and simple miracles.

I first met Olga in 1972, and we were close friends
until her death in 1985. A year and a half before her death,
I founded the Ambrose and Olga Worrall Institute of
Spiritual Healing. Ambrose, her husband, had for thirty-
five years worked with her in spiritual healing at Mount
Washington United Methodist Church in Baltimore. Each
Thursday morning, they performed spiritual healing on
more than three hundred people. Thousands of letters
from grateful patients arrived after the Worralls cured
their illnesses. Those letters are now at the Worrall Institute in Springfield, Missouri, with other mementos of their
work.

In 1975 I visited Olga at a healing service. A professor
of physics from Cleveland, Ohio, was there with a breast
cancer eroding through the skin of her breast; when I
examined her, the wound was black, swollen, and angry.
A month later, this educated woman sent a letter declaring
herself to be totally healed. Although in this case I have no
personal follow-up proof, there is little reason to doubt the
letter, especially in view of hundreds of other such reports.

Perhaps the most striking miracle of spiritual healing
I've ever seen was the cure of a woman with a malignant
brain tumor. After spiritual healing, her tumor disappeared. She had been through surgery without success,
and the experts had given her nine to eighteen months to
live. Four years later she was alive and well, with no
evidence of a brain tumor.

I have wanted, for many years, to collect adequate proof from physicians' records of at least twenty-five such miraculous healings. Interestingly, even when I have had letters from patients giving me permission to obtain their medical records, more than 99% of their physicians have failed to respond to my inquiry. I do, however, have medical records on ten patients in which miraculous "cures" occurred suddenly after spiritual healing, with no medical treatment.

In one sense, the healings of A.Z. and C.X., mentioned in the last chapter, were personally induced spiritual healing. The broad extent of spiritual healing is, however, adequately documented in many other examples, some going well beyond the laws of nature as we understand them.

Olga was able, for instance, to "heal" trypsin, an enzyme produced in the stomach to digest protein. Sister Justa Smith, a biochemist with a Ph.D., first damaged the trypsin physically. Olga laid hands on the test tubes of the trypsin and healed it, restoring its ability to digest protein. This accomplishment was well-documented by Sister Justa Smith. In experiments conducted by a physics professor, she healed bacteria on a culture plate that had been treated with an antibiotic, which would otherwise have killed them. Still other researchers recorded movements inside a closed cloud chamber when Olga sent healing energies from hundreds of miles away.

In 1977, Olga came to our clinic, joined by Dr. Elmer and Mrs. Alyce Green and other staff from the Menninger

Foundation, with elaborate recording equipment. With
Olga and Alyce in one room, Olga was hooked up with
sensors set to record skin resistance, pulse, and respiration,
as well as an EEG to measure brain activity and an EKG
to monitor her heart. Alyce held a microphone. Between
their room and a room holding Elmer Green with his staff
and recording equipment was an empty room. Another
empty room followed, and in the fifth room down the hall
lay a patient wired for EEG, EKG, pulse, skin resistance,
and respiration. I waited in that room with an "event"
marker to alert the recording equipment whenever I
observed changes in the patient.

Over the course of several days, Olga sent healing
messages to a total of twelve patients. In four of the twelve,
as Olga was sending her healing, the patients experienced
EKG, pulse, respiration, and/or EEG changes. One patient went into a deep trance, extending his head and neck,
with eyes closed but fluttering, exactly at the time Olga
started healing. The patient said, "I felt as if the aurora
borealis went off inside my head." His back pain vanished.

Another patient who had suffered from severe facial
pain for twenty-two years, unsuccessfully treated with
surgery and drugs, experienced complete relief of his pain
in a dream the evening of Olga's healing. Letters from his
wife and daughter two years later assured me that he
remained free of pain.

There are, of course, many varieties of spiritual
healing. In 1976, I spent two weeks in the Philippines with

Alyce and Elmer Green and a television film crew visiting seven psychic surgeons. Often three cameras, as well as three observers, watched proceedings from six different close-up angles. Some of the episodes were presented in a nationally broadcast film, "Psychic Phenomena–Exploring the Unknown," with Burt Lancaster, seen initially by twenty-eight million Americans on October 31, 1977. Several highlights of the Philippines trip are worth reporting.

In one situation, Tony Agpoa said, "Well, Norman, we do these materializations just to get the patient's belief system going." With that, he moved his hands on the abdomen of a woman, and I saw what appeared to be an open surgical wound with intestines visible through the peritoneum. I bent down beside the patient and saw that an image of the wound was floating about a half-inch above her abdomen. Tony then said, "Just as we can materialize, we can dematerialize." Without his moving his hands, I saw the image disappear. Tony had on a short-sleeved shirt, so no concealment was possible. I was allowed to follow him for the entire day, even into the men's room, and I was allowed to look under mattresses and anywhere I wished. I estimate that Tony removed more than two or three pints of blood that day; they were apparently materializations of blood. I was allowed to collect samples, and in every instance, it was human blood.

Another psychic surgeon, Tony Alcantra, performed

spiritual operations in a room about ten feet square, with cameras trained through the window and doors and with us observers close beside. Tony put his hands onto the abdomen of a woman with bladder cancer. Tony was in deep trance, with his eyes rolled up into his head and fluttering beneath his lids. More than a cup of blood and clots splattered all over the room, like popcorn gone wild. Again, pathology confirmed human blood, not animal blood, as some have claimed.

One of the most dramatic cases was with another healer who placed his hands on the neck of a person helping with the video taping. About two ounces of pus poured out as if an abscess had been opened with a knife, followed by a few drops of blood. This looked exactly like similar events in an operating room, and I know of no way to fake such pus, especially with the slight mixture of blood only at the end of the drainage. This was a miracle visually recorded for TV.

In another dramatic situation, a different healer removed at least two handsful of foul-smelling, sulphurous, rotten material from a woman on whom he claimed there had been a hex. It is impossible to understand where such foul material could have been hidden without evidence of sleight of hand being captured on three cameras or by three scientific observers. The laws of nature do not cover any aspect of such an experience.

Even more convincing was the visit of June Labo, one of the Philippine healers, to my clinic in September 1977.

June operated on some seventeen patients. In two cases I was able to collect samples of the surgically removed blood and compare it with blood I drew from the arm of that same patient. I also drew blood from June Labo. I personally took the blood samples to a forensic pathologist in Oakland, California, who confirmed that the blood from June was different and that the blood removed by June was identical to the individual patients' blood I had drawn. So I know for sure that no fakery took place.

In all these cases, it appeared as if the blood came *through* the skin. There was no apparent opening of the skin; blood just pooled, welling up around June's hands. Again, there is no law of nature to explain these phenomena. Although these materializations are in themselves not evidence of healing, they are clearly evidence of unexplainable miracles.

Many questions remain around the subject of spiritual healing. Why does it not occur more commonly? Like the placebo response, does it require the patient's belief? One answer may be found in a study done at a hospital in the United States. One group of patients was subjected, unbeknownst to them, to prayer healing, while a similar group served as controls without prayer. The group who received prayer had a statistically significant better recovery rate![1] At least some healing therefore occurs without any placebo. Is this grace? Why some heal and others fail to heal is as much an enigma as the unique healings that do occur.

There are two other facets of spiritual healing that, frankly, I rejected until early 1983, when I came suddenly face to face with challenges. I was doing a past-life therapy demonstration with seven students observing. Within a few minutes, I was dealing not with a past life but with a self-proclaimed demon. Even though I had never witnessed an exorcism, I had read enough and had enough presence of mind to proceed with this exorcism. I felt ecstatic when this event was concluded, and the student was freed of a virtual life-long depression, confirmed at follow-up six months later.

Shortly thereafter another patient, unaware of the event that morning, approached me with his sense of fear about the future. He could not see himself alive two years hence. Exploring this with him in a light trance, I encountered his mother's "energy" or personality. I encouraged the mother to leave and go on her own spiritual evolution. Seven years earlier on the night his mother had died, the student had felt ripped open and as if a cold breeze blew through him. He had been depressed for seven years. During his trance, when I addressed his mother, the patient's depression lifted instantly and at follow-up two years later, he remains free of depression.

Prior to these two experiences, I had assumed such events were evidence of hysteria but in neither of these patients was there any suspicion of hysteria. Since then, in one other student and three patients, I have had similar experiences of unexpected encounters with dark or evil forces, requiring exorcism. Meanwhile, I asked for and received consecration by a Catholic priest, Father Ron Roth, to sanctify such work.

In December 1993, I invited Father Ron to join me in evaluating ten patients who had not only failed all conventional medical approaches but who also had been unable to benefit from Biogenics training. In five of these individuals, we were able to evoke evidence of obsession with negative thought forms, but no other "possession." And despite efforts by Ron and me, no progress was made in any of these difficult patients.

Similarly, despite reports by a respected physician colleague from Kansas City that a shaman who did "soul retrieval" often successfully healed his difficult patients, four of my patients who had been consistent failures of therapy failed to benefit from the two-hour healing ceremony.

Another healer who reports many cures has been unsuccessful in healing four of my most recalcitrant patients. For twenty-plus years, I have been more concerned about the approximately 30% of my patients who fail to improve long-term. At least half of these unsuccessful patients did improve initially with two weeks of intense Biogenics retraining, often coupled with a variety of physical approaches.

My colleague, Caroline Myss, has addressed the issue of why people don't heal from her intuitive insight position. Rarely, the problem seems to be one of Karma–

unfinished business from a past life. Occasionally, she perceives that the patient has a personal sacred contract to go through a painful experience as a soul-gift to someone else. Caroline and I will be writing a whole book on sacred contracts. It is our belief that, before we are born, we make a contract at the soul level to work to develop particular spiritual skills, such as forgiveness or tolerance. Thus, at a soul level one may agree to go through birth as a deformed child to assist the parents in their own spiritual growth. Gladys McCarey in her wonderful book, *Born to Live,* recounts several examples of such soul-gifts.

Most often, however, such situations seem to be the result of a major spiritual crisis, one of inadequate will to overcome the emotional quagmire in which that person has become enmeshed. An inability or unwillingness to forgive someone else often appears to be the situation there. Forgiveness produces miracles; lack of forgiveness inhibits miracles.

Some individuals actually are so spiritually out of balance that they consciously decide to maintain their maladaptation. One thirty-year-old woman contacted me for assistance in applying for a compensation payment for health complications from her silicone breast implants. Actually, she had few symptoms, none that I could be certain had anything to do with her implants, and she assured me there was no way she would consent to removal of the implants. Despite the fact that many women complain about the preoccupation of men with size of their penis, my experience with at least fifty women who had breast implants suggests that at least some women have similar problems with their breasts. Surely, severe psychological concerns about the body are part of an existential or spiritual crisis. To these patients, even physical health is less important than their appearance.

Smoking can produce a similar problem. Despite the fact that 60% of the patients I see with severe chronic disease smoke—twice the average in all Americans—a striking majority of my patients refuse even to consider quitting the habit. Some admit they love smoking; others say it relaxes them; a few admit to being addicted. Some who even suffer from cancer of the lung refuse to quit smoking, even though it is known that five-year survival rates are twice as high for those who quit smoking once the diagnosis is made.

One twenty-eight year old woman suffering a severe connective-tissue disease, lupus, apparently resulting from or in association with silicone breast implants, was eager to have the implants removed but unwilling to quit smoking. I assured her that the symptoms of withdrawal could be easily controlled with nicotine skin patches and that a plastic cigarette could be used to address the habit portion. She was still unable to agree to try quitting tobacco, even though she acknowledged that it undoubtedly contributed to or aggravated her serious illness.

I see patients who hate their spouses with a passion and yet remain in totally unhappy, and sometimes dangerously abusive, relationships. Others hate their work or someone at work and are at least subconsciously unable to become well for fear of being forced back to a despised job or for fear of losing some unemployment pay.

A rare patient is clearly malingering, consciously faking symptoms and behavior in attempts to win large legal settlements. One such man pursued his multimillion-dollar suit despite extensive detective filming that showed him behaving totally normally in a myriad of situations when he was unaware of being filmed. In my opinion, his attorney, in assisting such a dishonest quest, was just as spiritually sick as he was.

Yes, Virginia, there are crooks! And these dishonest, sometimes dangerous, occasionally evil individuals make life hard for many others. M. Scott Peck has documented several such psychopathic situations, such as the parents who gave their twelve-year-old son the gun his older brother had used to commit suicide.[2]

In a similar way, many fundamentalist bigots provide outstanding examples of intolerance and hatred. Indeed, religious wars provide evidence that humanity has a long way to go to live the Golden Rule. Northern Ireland, the Middle East, Bosnia, Rwanda, and the Iraqi invasion of Kuwait are recent examples of the triumph of the opposite of spiritual healing. They are spiritual wounding at its deepest level.

Poverty, crime, war, rape, and murder are all evidence that life is not perfect. Virtually all the problems we see are created by people failing to live their lives in harmony with the one great Commandment, The Golden

Rule. And yet in the midst of such horrendous negativity, we find such great saints as Mother Teresa; the dedicated healers like Father Ron, Henry Rucker, and the Worralls, and the quiet, often unrecognized saints who deal with tragedy and deprivation with kindness, unconditional love and ever-present support. Love is, as in *The Urantia Book*, "The desire to do good to others."[3]

In 1982, as I finished a workshop in Indiana, a physician and his wife came up to share their experience. They told of a miraculous overnight cure of widespread cancer. The wife had been suffering for months with metastatic breast cancer, so prominent that lumps as big as her fist could be seen scattered over her body. One night she prayed that God either take her or heal her. The following morning she awoke, free of pain and the lumps. Now, five years later she remained free of cancer. Even though she did not report any attitudinal insight or change, and I have no medical records for her, I have no reason to question the veracity of this physician. Occasionally divine grace seems to provide sudden instant healing. My attitude towards these events is one of awe.

Ultimately, illness and suffering provide each of us the opportunity to choose our attitude, as Viktor Frankl so eloquently puts it in his epic work, *Man's Search for Meaning.* If you would have peace, embody the fruits of the spirit:

Forgiveness
Tolerance

Serenity

Compassion

Charity

Motivation

Joy

Faith

Hope

Confidence

Courage

Will

Reason

Wisdom

Love

And the greatest of these is Love.

With love all things are possible, including miracles. Forgiveness may be an essential beginning of the journey towards unconditional love.

As Caroline Myss has so profoundly taught, we come here with a sacred contract to use power responsibly, wisely, and lovingly. Spiritual healing, whether done by one through personal insight or achieved with the assistance of a spiritual healer, is one wise, responsible, and loving use of power.

And most recently, I have discovered a tangible, measurable result of spiritual healing. Paramount Studios sent a film crew to The Shealy Institute to record Henry Rucker performing spiritual healing. They wanted proof that something real took place. A fortunate intuitive insight led me to suggest measuring DHEA before and after healing. DHEA, dehydroepiandrosterone, is the most plentiful and most essential hormone in the human body. Healthy twenty-year-olds have blood levels of 900–1200 ng/dL. By age 80, most individuals are down to 130–180. And many adults with significant illnesses have great deficiencies of DHEA. Indeed, DHEA levels are unequivocal reflections of life energy reserves. Conventional medicine virtually ignores this crucial chemical because conventional medicine has no drugs to treat a deficiency of it.

Approximately an hour after Henry performed spiritual healing, blood levels of DHEA increased in three women by 22%, 55%, and 100%. Such miraculous changes in otherwise stable hormonal levels offer us proof that spiritual healing is real. In a later chapter, I shall offer my hypothesis of the energy laws that allow this phenomenon. At some point, I should like to see spiritual healings tested in this simple way. Of all the tests suggested to date, the effects on DHEA are perhaps the easiest to demonstrate. And since I consider DHEA to be the chemical equivalent of Life Force, DHEA may come closer to spirituality than hemoglobin or glucose.

In a study completed at a nursing home in Nuremberg, Germany, Professor Wolf Oswald, a psychologist, demonstrated that anyone who has a negative attitude toward age, sees no future for himself or herself, and has a passive outlook toward life "will age faster and stand a much poorer chance of survival." It appears that until we reach at least eighty-five years of age, "aging is mainly of our personal outlook on life and our social imprint."[4] Intelligence, on the opposite hand, doesn't peak until age forty or fifty. Old people who feel useless and unable to remedy the situation are cast aside into warehousing in nursing homes. Spiritual healing may be at its best in the elderly.

Spiritual healing may be the major factor in many alternative therapies. How does one distinguish spiritual healing from placebo? Ultimately, you can't. Why should spiritual healing be any different from aspirin or biofeedback? In most respects, I consider placebo to be spiritual healing. After all, it is belief or faith in something or someone. Expect healing, expect a miracle, and if your faith is great enough, then you have up to a 90% chance of success.

Obviously, there is a non-faith aspect to some healing, such as the healing of enzymes or bacteria, or the effect of absent prayer on coronary care patients when the patients did not know about the prayer. But the use of Qi Gong, a Chinese form of spiritual healing, and other meditative techniques is clearly related to spiritual healing. Even the Dean Ornish approach to coronary artery disease–diet, physical exercise and meditation–includes spiritual practice. Who knows the percentage of Ornish's success that is related to its spiritual component? From a conventional point of view, medicine would expect *prevention* of coronary disease with diet and physical exercise alone. But *reversal* of coronary atherosclerosis? Unlikely, yet contemporary physicians are still not rushing to recommend the Ornish program. Coronary angioplasty and bypass surgery haven't declined in popularity despite the safety and efficacy of this alternative approach. How sad!

And to which aspect of alternative healing does the following miracle case belong? In 1981 a fifty-one-year-old Catholic ex-priest came to me with severe angina pectoris and recommendations for coronary bypass surgery. He refused the operation. He had withdrawn from the priesthood a year and a half earlier and married an ex-nun. Our approach to his medical problem was a two-week educational program in Biogenics, our software program for self-regulation, and planned acupuncture to rebalance the energy of his heart. Shortly after I inserted the first needles, he passed out for about thirty seconds. When he awoke, he was free of angina, and within two weeks he was walking two miles free of pain. I hear from him from time to time. He remains symptom-free—a miracle in terms of medical expectations fourteen years ago. Was it the single acupuncture treatment, the stress reduction, or the ritual commitment to healing that improved his health?

Master Zheng Chen, who is seventy years old, says he healed himself of similar difficulties with Qi Gong, and there are many reports of miraculous healing with Qi Gong.

Are imagery and biofeedback ultimately ways of spiritual healing? I believe faith and expectation are critical factors in the potential for successful biofeedback therapy. Even hypnosis works ultimately through the power of the individual's focus of attention. Hypnosis simply allows the client to enter a state of focus in which positive suggestions are made part of the expectations, and thus faith or belief, of the individual. While these aspects of healing are less oriented toward God or Soul than is the laying on of hands or prayer, I consider all aspects of psychoneuroimmunology to be part of the spiritual aspect of life. Positive expectation is at the center of all spiritual practices and has as much to do with spirituality as the various religions have in common, namely the Golden Rule.

In 1958, during my year of surgical residency, a homeless, non-practicing Catholic woman who was a patient there developed tubercular pneumonia. She was considered terminal. A Catholic priest was called to give last rites. I stood in the door and refused to allow the priest in the room because I was convinced that last rites would be fatal to her minimal hope for recovery. The priest reluctantly performed last rites from the corridor. Only when my patient recovered did I share with her my intervention. She was most grateful and agreed that seeing a priest at that critical stage of her illness would have made it difficult for her to rally.

Was it my prayer, the almost-aborted hallway last rites, or synchronicity that allowed healing? Please do not misunderstand this case. I am not opposed to last rites of any religion; indeed, I believe in them fervently *if* the patient is comatose or *asks* for them. At the same time, I believe the meaning of last rites to a non-practicing Catholic who has not been in church for thirty years could be interpreted by that person as a death sentence.

Incidentally, I have routinely prayed for the healing of my patients, especially when I entered the operating room and for those who were critically ill. And I have often silently asked for divine healing to flow into patients when I hug or touch them. I suspect that at least some of the success of all medical/surgical intervention lies in the prayer of physicians, many of whom use prayer regularly.

As I stated earlier, spiritual healing is ultimately the foundation for the Body-Mind connection. As Ambrose Worrall so wisely stated, "Every thought is a prayer. It is evident, for instance, that a man must THINK, for he IS what he thinks. Thinking is what sets in motion spiritual forces to bring about the changes in his environment, his body, his companions, his language, his desires, his hopes, his despairs."[5]

Thinking is a spiritual practice. If your thoughts and prayers are to "create the condition desired," you should focus not on elimination of an undesired condition but upon the creation of healing. This is prayer and spiritual healing.

Although I have no personal experience with Tibetan

medicine, I have been consulted by a young man who told me he was cured by that method of treatment. This twenty-five-year-old man stated that he had had status asthmaticus for a year and a half, had seen leading asthma experts in the greater Boston area, had been placed on Prednisone, and was getting worse. He then consulted a Tibetan doctor, who gave him a variety of Tibetan herbs. Within one month he was totally cured. When he consulted with me, his asthma was no longer a problem, but he was moderately depressed. Nevertheless, the miracle of curing his asthma with a Tibetan herbal preparation is certainly not something we could expect in conventional medicine. Is this a form of spiritual healing or is it unresearched biochemistry?

Dr. Larry Dossey has emphasized the importance of prayer in healing yet medical journals generally refuse to publish studies on healing. In fact, Dr. George Lundberg, editor of the *Journal of the American Medical Association*, has stated, "We have received papers in this field (prayer), but I do not recall any paper making it past peer review." He goes on to state that they accept only "serious, scientific studies."[6]

NOTES

1. Larry Dossey, M.D., *Healing Words: The Power of Prayer and Practice of Medicine* (San Francisco: Harper San Francisco, 1993).

2. M. Scott Peck, *The Road Less Traveled* (New York: Simon and Schuster, 1978).

3. The Urantia Foundation, *The Urantia Book* (Chicago: Urantia Foundation, 1955).

4. *The German Tribune,* No. 1363 (March 19, 1989), p. 12.

5. Ambrose Worrall, "Essay on Prayer," March 1, 1952.

6. Editorial, *Wisconsin State Journal* (October 8, 1994), p. 1c.

Chapter 5

Acupuncture and GigaTENS

Miracles reflect
the laws of eternity,
not of time.
—A Course in Miracles

> Miracles arise from a
> miraculous state of mind,
> or a state of miracle readiness.
> *—A Course in Miracles*

Far more important than what the physician does
is the physician's belief and the patient's belief
in what the physician does.
—Sir William Osler, Father of American Medicine

Acupuncture has been used for thousands of years in

China to treat every illness imaginable. More than three hundred years ago, French Jesuit priests brought the technique of acupuncture to France, where it has undergone extensive scientific medical study and use. In the United States, acupuncture was used throughout the nineteenth century. In 1869 an American physician published the second edition of a volume on acupuncture.[1]

In 1912, Sir William Osler, the renowned medical historian, declared acupuncture to be the treatment of preference in lumbago, or low-back pain. He described the insertion of a solid needle into what acupuncturists would call Bladder 26.[2] I have seen miraculous instant cures of severe low-back pain with a single such treatment, which I have often performed since 1967.

The theory of acupuncture can be described fairly simply; and to me, a neurosurgeon with considerable experience in neurophysiology, the concept of acupuncture makes a great deal of sense. Indeed, nuclear physicists have recently confirmed the Chinese theory that each organ has a vector of vibratory energy projecting out from that organ, along the line of least resistance to a point at the tip of a finger or toe.[3] The energy is called Chi or Qi, Ki, prana, orgone energy, or life force. At one end point, this energy connects into the energy of a synchronous or harmonic path or meridian, thus completing a circuit. (Please see the acupuncture diagram on page 86.)

As in electricity, some energy is positive (yang) and some negative (yin). Both positive and negative energy are essential for life, and perfect balance between the positive and the negative is essential for health.

Here, in a nutshell, is the theory behind acupuncture: A small solid needle, which separates rather than cuts tissue, provides a tiny input of electrical energy to boost Chi. As in electricity, it is possible to have blocks, short circuits, areas of excess or deficient capacity or current. A small physical electrical boost may help reestablish normal flow and health–what Western science has called homeostasis, or balance.

It is certainly known that, normally, the autonomic nervous system provides the mechanism for homeostasis after the fight-or-flight stress response. And virtually all disease involves imbalance in autonomic function. To some extent, dysautonomia–problems with autonomic nerve function–represents electrically, physiologically confirmed evidence of electromagnetic disturbance, which apparently can be healed by the tiny electric currents provided by acupuncture. Dr. Irvin Korr described the problem as a "facilitated spinal segment," where a small injury *lowers the threshold* of nerve sensitivity so that electrical oversensitivity results.[4] Acupuncture appears to work at a more subtle level.

Thousands of Americans and Europeans have benefited from the resurgence of acupuncture as a treatment in the past twenty years, a resurgence initiated in 1972 when James Reston of the *New York Times* reported his post-appendectomy treatment. A number of scientific articles

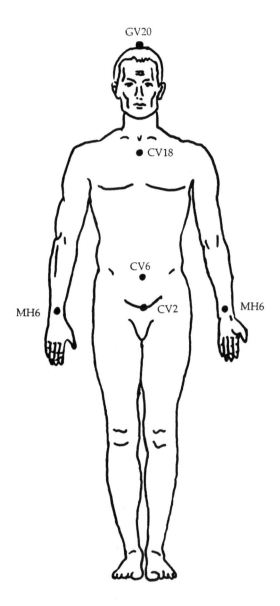

Illustration 1(a) and (b). Acupuncture points for the Ring of Fire. See pages 97–98 for explanation of acupuncture points.

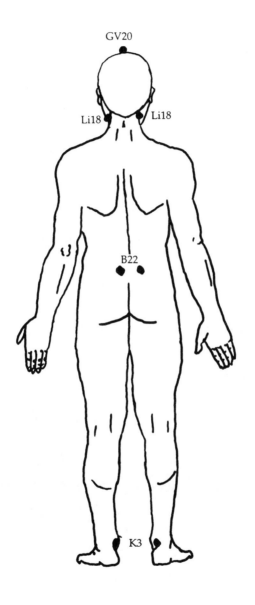

have documented clinical and laboratory changes with acupuncture, including such effects as increases in cortisone and beta endorphins. Despite the evidence that acupuncture is more effective than are 99% of drugs, American physicians and the insurance mafia still attack and malign acupuncture. Properly done, acupuncture is safer than any drug. Its major uses are in pain control, addiction, control of anxiety, and restoration of fertility in infertile males.

Pain Control

For both acute and chronic pain, acupuncture offers significant relief in about 80% of patients. This puts it on a par with morphine—without the risk of addiction or of side effects!

Here is a case in point. Sarah, the forty-five-year-old wife of a stockbroker, arrived at our clinic complaining of severe migraine at least weekly, the pain of which sometimes left her non-functional for three or four days. She received weekly acupuncture treatments for six weeks, every two weeks for two months, then monthly for a few months. She returns now about once a year for a "tune-up." She currently suffers only one or two migraines each year. She has resisted biofeedback training or counseling for her unsatisfying marriage but is still improved above 90% with a safe and remarkably effective treatment. Miraculous? Yes. No drug approach and no other intervention is this effective. She could probably be improved

100% if she would care for herself a bit more! And her response to acupuncture, contrary to the "laws" of allopathic medicine, is a miracle.

PMS

Dr. Joseph Helms has designed a treatment of PMS, premenstrual syndrome, that proved highly successful statistically, and he published his findings in the major gynecological journal. Yet in a peer-reviewed scientific journal he was still largely ignored.[5]

Dr. Helms's course in acupuncture for physicians began at our family's farm in 1979 and has grown to an annual student body of more than two hundred students, each receiving two hundred hours of Category I continuing education credit through UCLA, a course approved by the American Medical Association. This accomplishment in itself is almost a miracle.

Back Pain

I have already mentioned the remarkable effectiveness of acupuncture in back pain. In my opinion, everyone suffering significant back pain should try acupuncture for three treatments. If they are improved 50% or more, then the acupuncture is worth continuing. It is thousands of times safer than drugs or surgery and provides many more miracles!

Addiction Control

A number of physicians have demonstrated excellent addiction control with acupuncture. Dr. Richard Kroening, initially of UCLA, has been at the forefront in this approach.[6] When you consider the terrible failure of our expensive drug and alcohol rehabilitation programs in the United States, it is immoral and unethical to deny addicts acupuncture treatment. (Fortunately, in most European countries, acupuncture is more widely accepted and reimbursed.) At costs of $30,000 and more for a month of treatment, the one-year success rate of most drug programs is less than 10%. Even at a 50% cure rate, acupuncture offers a less expensive approach that has proved five times as successful. How long do we have to wait for scientific and common sense, as well as financial benefit, to require acupuncture treatment for drug and alcohol abuse?

Of great interest is the equally good use of cranial electrical stimulation and GigaTENS. But more about that later.

Anxiety

The Chinese have a treatment for "non-violent madness," or severe agitation. I have practiced it for more than twenty years, with remarkable success. Totally safe and less expensive than tranquilizers, the use of acupuncture in calming anxiety is as potent as physical exercise and deep relaxation. For the patient, it can seem miraculous. Compare the performance of acupuncture for agitation with that of tranquilizers! In fact, there is simply no situation in which I am willing to prescribe or recommend tranquilizers long-term. For some acute situations, they may be tried, but I believe they are the worst invention of modern conventional medicine and the one to be most avoided by intelligent people.

Male Infertility

Dr. M. Mussat, a renowned French physician, brought to my awareness the use of acupuncture in restoring fertility. Infertility affects about 30% of American males who are functionally sterile (who produce fewer than twenty million sperm). There is essentially no medical treatment for this emotionally and spiritually distressing condition.

I have published a paper confirming Dr. Mussat's observations in four patients. With only twelve treatments, one man's sperm count rose from twelve million to fifty-four million.[7] One happy miracle!

Acupressure

Acupressure is the use of firm, slightly painful pressure, usually with a thumb or knuckle over appropriate acupuncture points. For most headaches, acupressure is safe and more effective than aspirin or any other drug. Pressure is applied on both sides at Bladder 10, the lateral bone of the second cervical vertebra, located at the nape of the neck; at Large Intestine 4; or at Hoku, the tender point in the center of the muscle between thumb and index finger.

Sometimes pressure needs to be reapplied three or

four times, but within two to three minutes, near miraculous relief can be achieved. Everyone should learn this technique. Acupressure may be helpful for a variety of other pains and problems. Look for books on acupressure and Do-In.

TENS

In 1966, when I began trying dorsal column stimulation, it seemed to me that I had to have some way of demonstrating to prospective patients the potential sensation of electrical stimulation. I reached into my memory for an old device, patented in 1919 by a naturopath, C. W. Kent, and given to my father by a chiropractor many years earlier to control a painful Bell's palsy or facial paralysis. Conventional medicine had nothing to offer him, but this device, the Electreat, allowed him complete pain relief and recovery of movement.

Although a bit cumbersome, the Electreat proved to be more than a test device; it actually helped thousands of patients. I pleaded with biomedical engineers for about seven years to make a more modern, solid-state electrical stimulator; finally, I succeeded. Today there are dozens of types of transcutaneous electrical nerve stimulation (TENS) devices in use in virtually every civilized country in the world. Interestingly, I have maintained for twenty years that Electreat is better than the modern TENS devices. Later, I'll share with you the recent proof of my assertion.

Properly used, TENS is totally safe and controls pain

in 80% of cases of acute pain and helps greatly in 50% of patients with chronic pain. It should be the first treatment of choice in virtually every significant pain problem. Indeed, in most countries it is available over-the-counter, even in department stores, at a cost of a quarter to an eighth of our prescription-required and delinquently prescribed ones in the United States. At this point, at least hundreds of thousands (it should be millions) of patients have received benefit from TENS. If you or a loved one has pain and has not yet had adequate trial of TENS, demand it. And if your physician won't or can't provide it, find another physician!

GigaTENS

In 1925, Georges Lakhovsky published in France his book, *The Secret of Life*. In 1935, it was translated into English, but it has been systematically ignored by scientists.[8] Lakhovsky stated that DNA of human cells vibrates at fifty billion cycles per second. In the late 1930s, he moved to the United States. Soon reports of several hundred cures of a variety of serious illnesses, including cancer, came from a New York hospital! Unfortunately, Lakhovsky was killed in a motor vehicle accident in 1941, and no further work on his oscillator has been available in this country.

The Lakhovsky multiwave oscillator is triggered by a Tesla coil or violet ray, a high-frequency electrical device frequently recommended by Edgar Cayce for treatment of a variety of conditions, even for restoring hair on a bald head. And indeed, it does work, at least as well as Rogaine! Rogaine, incidentally, restores hair well about 11% of the time, moderately 11% of the time, and just a bit 11% of the time, at a cost of about $60 per month forever. For $135, one can instead purchase a violet ray, and it is safe except for someone with a cardiac pacemaker. However, don't use it in the room with a modem telephone or computer! For more details on the violet ray, consult the Association for Research and Enlightenment (A.R.E.) in Virginia Beach, Virginia.

In 1992 I was invited to visit the Ukraine to evaluate a treatment called Microwave Resonance Therapy. I spent a hundred hours in classroom and clinical education there learning about this treatment. According to Ukrainian nuclear physicists, the DNA of human cells vibrates at from fifty-two to seventy-eight billion cycles per second, at a power intensity of a billionth of a watt. Plant DNA vibrates at forty-two billion cycles per second (or GigaHertz, GHz); animal DNA vibrates at forty-seven GHz. The sun produces all known frequencies in the electromagnetic field, including fifty-two to seventy-eight GHz at one ten-billionth of a watt/cm^2 of space. We thus live in a bath of GHz. See the Insight Meditation Chamber described in the Chapter 9. It is a simple amplifier of GHz.

Ukrainian quantum physicists believe each of us may have an optimal or unique frequency, such as 62.422268 GHz. This vibration, just as does an EEG or EKG, is reflected out to the surface of the body along the acupuncture meridians described by the Chinese. In illness, the amplitude is diminished in an appropriate meridian. By using one-billionth of a watt of energy at fifty-two to seventy-eight GHz for thirty minutes, five days a week for two weeks, many illnesses can be cured or put into remission for many months.

At the time of our visit, the nuclear physicists had treated two hundred thousand patients with almost every known illness. Their greatest success was in treating immune dysfunctions, of which they had many, because of the Chernobyl accident only sixty miles from Kiev. They showed us very sophisticated immune studies demonstrating marked improvements with GigaTENS therapy. I have chosen to call this therapy GigaTENS because it most closely resembles a subtle transcutaneous electrical nerve stimulator, and indeed the Electreat puts out GHz activity–similar in many ways to the Ukrainian devices. This is why the Electreat is better than most TENS devices!

In Kiev, endocrinologists, diabetologists, cardiologists, and orthopedists are all enthusiastic about GigaTENS. Most striking is the 50% long-term success rate in treating narcotic addiction (just ten treatments) and 56% success with alcoholics. In fact, if they can get to the alcoholic to begin treatment just at the stage after drying out, when the alcoholic craves a drink, their success rate goes up to 90%! The potential cost effectiveness of this treatment is mind-boggling. But as with all innovations, it may be twenty or thirty years before GigaTENS is accepted here in the United States. After all, TENS, grudgingly and limitedly accepted here, is still prescribed inadequately. A strong part of me wishes we were as free as patients in many other countries, where such treatments are at least available over-the-counter for those wise enough to use them.

Our preliminary results at the Shealy Institute in chronic back pain, rheumatoid arthritis, depression, and diabetic neuropathy are all promising. I expect to continue developing research with GigaTENS for the next five years or more. At this time, one of the most promising is the possibility of restoring dehydroepiandrosterone (DHEA) production. If this is substantiated, GigaTENS will offer the most exciting miracle of all alternatives: the potential for rejuvenation and even for regrowth of limbs and the spinal cord.

The concept of solar acupuncture, which is beyond the known laws of nature, has the potential for leading us to new laws! It may some day no longer be a miracle, but today it remains only the brightest star on the horizon.

THE RING OF FIRE

In three individuals we have increased DHEA, my favorite hormone, by 49% and 60% simply by using only GigaTENS on the circuit of the body I call the Ring of Fire. This is the first demonstration of increasing DHEA by a simple, safe technique. If I can replicate this effect in even half of those lacking in this hormone, GigaTENS will become the most successful, powerful tool ever discovered. It has the potential for miraculously healing otherwise incurable problems.

As noted in the chapter on spiritual healing, the increases in DHEA with Henry Rucker's spiritual healing suggest that he is able to serve as a channel or amplifier of GHz available from the sun. In GigaTENS we may thus be seeing the first evidence of electrically assisted spiritual healing. Is it possible that Henry and other healers simply serve as antennae/transmitters for cosmic Energy?

CAROLINE MYSS AND THE RING OF FIRE

Caroline Myss and I have theorized that the Ring of Fire is the essential battery of the body. This core energy system maintains and coordinates Chi, Qi, Ki, prana, orgone energy, or life force—whatever you choose to call it. In every known culture, the concept of a universal energy is considered essential to life. Although the Chinese described many circuits of energy, they did not include the Ring of Fire. As we see it, the human battery consists of the connection of pineal and pituitary through windows of the sky to master of the heart, which is the control center for the autonomic and sympathetic system, through the thyroid gland, adrenal glands, testicles or ovaries, uterus or prostate, to the kidneys. The acupuncture points I have chosen are:

GV 20 • top center of the head

Li 18 • one inch below the tip of the mastoids, between sternocleidomastoid and trapezius muscles

MH 6 • the point about one inch above the center
of the front of each wrist

CV 18 • an inch below the sternal notch

B 22 • one inch lateral to the center of the spine
at the second lumbar vertebra

CV 6 • about an inch below the umbilicus or
belly button

CV 1 • at the center of the perineum, between
the anus and genitalia

K 3 • inside the ankles, in the hollow

At this time, we have demonstrated that stimulation of
these points cumulatively for thirty minutes, using the
GigaTENS or the Liss Cranial Electrical Stimulator, can
increase DHEA significantly.

Interestingly, natural progesterone cream, 3%,
ProGest, also increases DHEA from 50 to 100%. For
restoration of DHEA in individuals with levels below the
optimal of 750 ng/dL in men or 550 ng/dL in women, I
recommend the following treatment.

Twelve Steps to Rejuvenating Your Ring of Fire

1. Expose yourself to natural light. Be outside
   without glasses at least one hour every day.
   Eight hours would be ideal.

2. Engage in physical exercise. Earn sixty aerobics
   points per week.

3. Use the Liss cranial electrical stimulator on Ring of Fire points thirty minutes every day.*

4. Apply ProGest cream (available from Self-Health Systems, 5607 South 222nd Road, Fair Grove, MO 65648), 1/4 tsp. twice a day. In men apply to the scrotum and inside thighs. In women, apply to breasts and inside thighs.

5. Be happy! Perform a laughing meditation fifteen minutes twice a day. A laughter tape is available from Self-Health Systems.

6. Resolve your anger, guilt, anxiety, and depression. See Chapter 3 on self-regulation.

7. Use magnets, with north pole towards the Ring of Fire points, while meditating daily on the Ring of Fire. A tape is available from Self-Health Systems.

8. Use a music bed daily with great music, as discussed in Chapter 9 on depression.

9. Massage the Ring of Fire points, with the intent to strengthen it, or stoke the fire!

10. Minimize air travel and exposure to electro-magnetic contamination.

11. Minimize sugar, caffeine, and alcohol.

12. Eat real foods in great variety.

---

* The combination of Liss CES, GigaTENS, and ProGest is so unique that a patent application for the process has been filed.

If you are a woman, and your DHEA is below 130 ng/dL or a man and below 180 ng/dL, I recommend DHEA supplementation for at least three months while using the above twelve-step program. Men should try 25 mg. four times a day and recheck their DHEA in two weeks. If it's not at 750 ng/dL they should increase the dose to achieve 750 ng/dL. A woman should aim for 550 ng/dL. After three months, they should wean themselves from the treatment over a two-week period, continuing the twelve-step DHEA program. On the final day and the day after stopping DHEA supplementation, they should have injections of ACTH 25 mg. and Factrel 500 micrograms. They should recheck their DHEA the following day, then continue working on all levels until the optimal DHEA levels have been reached. You cannot afford adrenal/Chi depletion.

If, after undergoing the above program you cannot restoke your reserves, it is probably advisable to stay on DHEA supplementation. To engage in the program you will need a cooperating physician. Considering the difficulty we have encountered in getting TENS widely used, we are currently exploring the possibility of establishing DHEA restoration programs throughout the world.

NOTES

1. A.R. Brown, M.D., *Treatise on Acupuncturation,*

Inoculation, Diversion, and Direct Medical Administration (Albion, MI: Published by A.R. Brown, 1869).

2. Sir William Osler, *The Principles and Practice of Medicine,* 8th ed. (Chicago: Daniel Appleton and Co., 1912).

3. Dr. Norman Shealy, personal visit to Kiev, January 1993.

4. *The Collected Papers of Irvin M. Korr,* ed. B. Peterson (Newark, OH: American Academy of Osteopathy, 1979).

5. C. Norman Shealy, M.D.; Joseph Helms, M.D.; and Allen McDaniels, M.D., "Treatment of Male Infertility with Acupuncture," *The Journal of Neurological and Orthopaedic Medicine and Surgery* 11 (December 1990): 285–286.

6. R. J. Kroening and T.D. Oleson, "Rapid Narcotic Detoxification in Chronic Pain Patients Treated with Auricular Electroacupuncture and Naloxone," *International Journal of Addictions* 9 (1985): 1347–1360.

7. Shealy, Helms, and McDaniels, "Treatment of Male Infertility with Acupuncture."

8. Georges Lakhovsky, *The Secret of Life: Electricity, Radiation, and Your Body,* 4th ed. (Costa Mesa, CA: Noontide Press, 1988).

Chapter 6

Chiropractic and Osteopathy: Body Therapy

To adjust or to manipulate—
that is the question.
—*Hamlet* (paraphrased)

Just over a hundred years ago, Andrew Taylor Still, a Missouri physician, rediscovered an ancient technique: manipulation to restore health. Even though allopathy had little to offer at that time, the medical profession totally rejected this important therapeutic tool. Indeed, for at least six decades the AMA fought osteopathy tooth and nail. Then in an abrupt turnaround in the mid 1960s, the AMA suddenly "accepted" osteopaths (D.O.s) as "equal" in training to M.D.s. Doctors of Osteopathy were offered an opportunity to become M.D.s overnight. In doing so, the AMA was apparently hoping to abolish osteopathy. But fortunately some wiser minds prevailed, refusing to give up their unique approach to illness. Unfortunately, most D.O.s subsequently trained, in order to seem part of the crowd, gave up their uniqueness and failed to learn how to manipulate the body.

Still's major thesis was that relatively minor abnormalities of position, especially of the vertebrae, led to constriction of blood vessels. The resultant relative loss of blood flow, and thus oxygen, led to malfunction of affected organs.

Within a few years of Still's beginning his School of Osteopathic (pathology of the bones or skeleton) Medicine, D.D. Palmer apparently visited Still for two weeks as a patient. Palmer had been a fish salesman in his hometown of Davenport, Iowa. About six months after he visited Still, Palmer began the study of chiropractic (practice with the hands). He insisted that "subluxations" of the spine were compressing nerve roots, and that the resultant loss of nerve energy led to organ pathology. Instead of manipulating the skeleton manually, Palmer "adjusted" it.

Within a few years, B.J. Palmer, son of the founder of chiropractic who also used it, split with his more eclectic father, and two major chiropractic visions ensued: the "straights" of B.J. Palmer, who insist that adjustment is the only legitimate treatment for virtually every illness, and the "mixers" who incorporate such approaches as nutrition, vitamin/mineral supplements, herbs, and hydro and electrotherapy. In fact, in twelve states mixers are also taught minor surgery and obstetrics.

Because of allopathy's rejection of manipulation or adjustment, many miracles have been performed by manual therapists. Of course, these are miracles only because allopathic medicine refuses to accept the simple proof of the principles of spinal misalignment.

My first encounter with chiropractic came in 1966 when I walked down some stairs with a bag of concrete and leaned over to pour it into the foundation for a swing set. I suddenly couldn't stand up. For two weeks, I walked around bent and twisted and in pain. I felt as if my sacroiliac joint was stuck. Finally, I approached an orthopedist and asked him to manipulate my back. I sensed, knowing nothing about such procedures, that a good brisk jerk would get me moving again. The orthopedist (straight foot, indeed!) refused, declaring, "That's witchcraft!"

Reluctantly and untrustingly, I made an appointment to see Dr. Howard Barge, on the recommendation of a neighbor. I refused to allow an x-ray; I asked him just to adjust my sacroiliac. One simple, fast, and very short movement, a tiny "pop," and I got off the table straight and free of muscle spasm and pain. From an allopathic point of view, this "witchcraft" produced a welcome miracle!

Shortly thereafter, I was the medical society's volunteer to campaign for fluoridation of the water supply of La

Crosse, Wisconsin. I had swallowed that bit of allopathic ignorance; after all, most dentists pushed for fluoridation. I didn't realize that even then a few wiser dentists did not. The campaign was bitter. Every naturalist attacked me and the medical profession. Full-page ads with skull and crossbones accused me of being a murderer. The opposing campaign was led by Dr. Fred Barge, nephew of Dr. Howard Barge. Fred Barge and some lay persons flooded my mailbox with letters and literature. I began to realize that there was some excellent evidence that fluoride was indeed a poison and that cumulatively, at best, it is not good for you. Fred's campaign prevailed, and he invited me to lunch. For the next fifteen years, he educated me about the benefits of chiropractic.

Over that fifteen-year period, Dr. Fred Barge sent me many more patients with physical neurosurgical diseases than any doctor in town! Probably through both intuition and skill, Fred recognized brain and spinal cord tumors and truly ruptured discs that had been missed by M.D.s. About a year later I leaned over in my garden on a Saturday afternoon and couldn't straighten up. I phoned Fred and asked, "Are you going to your office tomorrow?" Of course he agreed to see me, and once again I experienced the wonderful miracle of instant cure with a simple adjustment. At least a dozen times I had recurrent sudden catches in my back, with just as rapid cure by Fred's hands. I once told him he'd be out of business if all his patients recovered so quickly.

Gradually, Fred revealed to me some remarkable cases in which scoliosis was corrected, changes impossible to achieve according to the blind laws of allopathy. Then, in the late 1970s when my daughter developed a mild scoliosis, and after an orthopedist recommended a brace, I took her instead to Fred. Over the course of a year, with perhaps two dozen adjustments and an exercise program, Laurel recovered. I can only wonder how many miracles have been missed by allopathy's rejection of spinal adjustment. Not only are miracles missed, but great tragedies are produced when teenagers are placed in braces and large segments of their spines are crudely fused. They remain cursed with rigid, painful spines. Indeed, today I urge anyone with early scoliosis to find a competent chiropractor or osteopath to assist in recovery. And, of course, there are now electrical stimulators that can assist the process of muscle balancing so essential to improvement in scoliosis.

In 1973, on my second visit to the A.R.E. at Virginia Beach, Virginia, Dr. Genevieve Haller introduced me to Dr. O. Raymond Simpson, a retired chiropractor in his late seventies, who in five minutes diagnosed a dislocated first rib as the cause of my eighteen-year history of right suprascapular pain. He performed the most remarkable and simple adjustment of my rib, and for three days the pain was miraculously gone. After that, a dull and relatively minor return of pain occurred. Still, the miracle of sudden relief, and indeed permanent and major improvement, left me in awe of his skill.

Even though I had never met an osteopathic physician, in 1978 when I founded the American Holistic Medical Association I knew that I wanted an osteopath on the founding board. Fortunately for me, Dr. Jerry Dickey joined early. At first he wondered what my ulterior motives were in asking him to become an officer of AHMA.

Jerry introduced me to the wide variety of osteopathic manipulative techniques: high velocity, low amplitude; low velocity, high amplitude; strain-counter-strain; muscle energy; and cranial osteopathy. And my education expanded to understand the science of osteopathy.

One of the great researchers in spinal physiology, Dr. Irvin M. Korr, known as Kim, published scores of excellent research papers, demonstrating the multifactorial response of the spinal cord to minor mechanical problems. Kim's brilliant demonstration of the "facilitated spinal segment" remains one of the great ignorances of allopathy. Such "minor" abnormalities as an eighth of an inch of difference in leg length can put a postural strain on one or more vertebrae, resulting in electrical hyperactivity of the spinal cord in that segment. Muscle spasm and a variety of electrical and vascular abnormalities ensue.[1]

Kim also demonstrated both organ dis-ease from spinal dysfunction and spinal dysfunction resulting from muscle spasm, created reflexly by organ pathology! It's a two-way street, one system affecting the other negatively.

Pancreatitis (inflammation of the pancreas), for instance, created by a gallstone lodged in the bile duct–

which crosses the pancreas—can lead to severe thoracic back pain and spinal misalignment from the reflex paraspinal muscle spasm.

Conversely, a fall or sudden twist, which leads to spinal facet locking, causes paraspinal muscle spasm and pain. The resultant electrical disturbance can influence the pancreas to create pancreatitis. Is it any wonder that physicians have difficulty finding the cause of such an illness? Especially when the great majority of physicians don't know this simple fact? Or even how to examine the spine adequately!

It appears that Still and Palmer were both right. Spinal subluxations can "pinch" either nerves or arteries, with resulting possible electrical dysfunction. Ultimately, the head bone is connected to the tail bone and everything in between.

And speaking of the head bone: cranial osteopathy offers the most remarkable example of an enigma. According to allopathy, the skull in an adult is immobile. Having operated scores of times on the skull, I'd never seen the bones move. But good osteopaths and clever chiropractors believe that the individual bones never totally fuse. At those little squiggly interdigitations, they say, the bones move, not up and down, but essentially from side to side.

In 1979 Dr. John Upledger was visiting me. John is a very talented osteopathic physician. A twenty-five-year-old private patient I'd never seen before was brought by

his father to see me because of total incapacity following
a skiing accident two years earlier. The young man suffered from what were essentially constant headaches. At
least fourteen M.D.s had failed to find a cause or cure for
the headaches. Skull and spine films, CAT scans, EEG,
and neurologic exams were all normal.

As the young man entered my office, he lunged for
me, furious at seeing another "stupid" doctor. The father
and John Upledger stopped him. John suggested he examine the patient's head. He spent perhaps fifteen minutes
and performed a simple cranial manipulation. The young
man, smiling and free of headache, apologized! John did
another gentle osteopathic manipulation just for good
measure, and the young man went home cured by this
miracle.

Three years later he dropped by my office when I
moved to Missouri to thank me for his cure; it was John
Upledger, of course, who performed the cure. Again, I
wonder how many suffering patients continue to fail
multiple drug and psychological treatments because physicians remain ignorant of these safe alternatives.

In 1985, while doing simple stretching exercises I'd
done hundreds of times, I suddenly caught my sacroiliac.
I was on a trip at the time, but fortunately I was returning
home that evening. The pain in my left buttocks and sciatic
nerve was as severe as a fractured hip had been fourteen
years earlier. By the following morning, there was a
swelling the size of my index finger along the top side of

my left foot, coupled with numbness. Three osteopathic physicians worked on me, the last finally getting my sacral shear back in place. The pain was gone instantly and the swelling and numbness subsided over the next week. A significant miracle in allopathic terms!

I have since learned to diagnose and treat such rotations of the sacrum—major causes of low back and sciatic pain in about 15% of chronic back pain problems. Each of these patients has been misdiagnosed by several to a dozen M.D.s who have often operated inappropriately on a bulging, non-ruptured disc. Such patients are told eventually, "Nothing is wrong; it's all in your head." Each has the potential, with appropriate manipulation, for miraculous cure.

There are, of course, some pitfalls of manipulation of the spine, and occasionally some serious complications. But all the reported complications of spinal manipulation for the past hundred years will never equal the complications of almost any single drug, anesthetic or surgical procedure. The tragedy of allopathy's ignoring chiropractic and osteopathy is the lack of cooperation and cross-education among disciplines. Intelligent and wise evaluation of the mechanics of the spine would add more benefit to humanity than all the drugs of the world. But ignoring drugs and surgery, when they are needed, such as in meningitis or appendicitis, respectively, would be equally tragic. The bottom line is that neither field is optimal without the other.

In addition to chiropractic and osteopathy, patients have access to a number of other body therapies, ranging from the physical psychotherapy of Wilhelm Reich, a tragically rejected M.D. psychiatrist, to simple massages, Rolfing, Feldenkrais Therapy, Alexander Therapy, and many more. Each of these fields offers part of the whole potential for healing. Although I personally have few miracles to report in these diverse specialties, many therapists report great benefit with their approaches.

Although my evaluation of the work of Kay Ortmans is perhaps primarily psychological insight, she has provided me with some of the most miraculous experiences. I met Kay in the early 1970s. She developed a technique of slow, gentle body massage done to a background of moderately loud stereo classical music. She believes we store in our muscles memories of painful events from past lives–not the past of this life but past incarnations. In 1975, I invited Kay, after my earlier experience of her talent, to come to my clinic for a week.

I introduced Kay to the patients as a good masseuse. She did her work, about two hours of kneading massage, on each of four patients. The instructions she gave them are simple: "Keep your mind focused on the music. If you have any images that seem important, you may share them with me." She gives no suggestion that the images might be those of the events a hundred years or more earlier! Each of the four patients, incredulous after their experience, explained to me their amazement at the images of a past life, each totally unexpected, each providing emotionally useful therapeutic insights into current problems.

I've had at least a dozen personal experiences with Kay. Perhaps the most striking occurred when she was working on the chronically tight area in my right suprascapular area, which was tender but not spontaneously painful since Dr. Simpson's work. After about an hour of steady work, Kay put Rachmaninoff's *Isle of the Dead* on her player and resumed massage of my upper back. I suddenly burst out laughing at the image I'd had. I saw myself being hanged, as a priest, because I was caught having sex with the bishop's daughter! I knew that, in this situation, it was okay for the bishop to have sex (and thus a daughter), but a lowly priest could not. The miracle here is the evocation of a powerful emotional image, one far more intense than any dream or fantasy I'd ever experienced.

Whether that past life actually took place is of no importance; the scenes are as clear to me today as is the paper on which this is written. Did I tune in, through Kay's stimulation, to an event recorded in the collective unconscious or the morphogenic field? Is Kay a channel similar to Henry Rucker, allowing my less-talented receiver (mind) access to the history of the world—or to myself?

The historical accuracy of the event is immaterial; the emotional impact of such experiences is sometimes more real than current life. I've observed Kay repeating this magic on many other people and teaching it to others. In

1982, she led a workshop at my clinic where the staff learned and experienced this powerful technique. During that weekend I had at least four almost equally vivid day "dreams." Is this memory stored in the body and released by simple muscle manipulation, or is it just a physiologic trigger into a REM (rapid eye movement) state in which the brain conjures up allegories? Certainly, I've never had such dreams at night. And during that same period each member of my staff had vivid memories that were unlike their usual dreams.

The simple postural work of Alexander provides a very different approach to health. An actor, F. Matthias Alexander, lost his voice and could not find relief from a number of physicians. Interestingly, Alexander was married to the daughter of an otolaryngologist, or ear, nose, and throat specialist. Eventually, Alexander learned that his posture was the cause of his dis-ease. Although he had no medical training, he discovered that many illnesses could be overcome with proper adjustment of posture.

The Alexander approach is as gentle as Rolfing is vigorous. An Alexander therapist simply places hands on areas of excess muscle tension with no pressure and encourages relaxation adequate to lead to proper posture. The session may include almost no talk and certainly includes no physical pressure. But the results can be striking. In my first Alexander session, a British osteopath who primarily does Alexander therapy placed his hands on my hips. As I stood in his office, I instantly realized that despite more than twenty years of deep relaxation training, as soon as I stood up I assumed the warrior position! I was totally tensed for fighting or fleeing. Immediately after that one-hour session, I walked straight for the first time in almost sixty years. I'd always been slew-footed, but after that treatment I felt as if I were floating as I effortlessly walked for three hours. More than two years later I still have to think about my posture and let go of useless tension that automatically returns each day. But the effort I make has decreased: the new habit is increasingly easier. And the memory of that miracle of a simple hand on my hip remains.

Rolfing, on the other hand, involves deep tissue massage, often painful, theoretically to release fascial restrictions. Fascia is the spider web-like material between muscles, the liquid glue that allows muscles to glide over one another.

Dr. Ida Rolf, a biochemist, came to her concept of Rolfing as intrinsically as all the other body therapists. Rolfers go over the entire body, slowly and deeply, pressing on restricted areas until the muscles release their iron-like grip. There are numerous anecdotes of clients having miraculous emotional insights during Rolfing. I have myself enjoyed perhaps sixty sessions over twenty years. Even though I've never had a miraculous insight during Rolfing, I've often felt the beta-endorphin high the day after a Rolfing session. Clearly, this technique leads to powerful neurochemical responses.

What do Rolf, Alexander, Still, and Palmer have in common? It appears that each of these innovators has lit a dark corner in the Cretan labyrinth of the physical body. Emotional stress leads to muscle tension and postural changes, sometimes quite marked. Trauma may also create postural misalignment, maintained by the reflex muscle spasm resulting from skeletal pain. And internal diseases reflexively cause protective muscle spasm. Ultimately, the mechanical postural muscular spasm alters physiology, electrically and chemically.

And there is the remarkable work of Dr. Dannanberg, a podiatrist who has demonstrated that many postural strains can be corrected with simple but proper orthotics. He showed me videos of patients whose multiple back surgeries had all failed, who were cured in five or ten minutes with insertion of a flexible soft insert into the shoes. The instant removal of long-standing pain by the change in posture correction appears to the patient and observer to be a miracle.

On a somewhat less esoteric note, there is the delightful work of the late Dr. Skyrme Rees, an Australian urologist turned neurosurgeon. In 1972, I attended the Pan Pacific Surgical Congress in Hawaii, primarily because I wanted a February vacation in a warm place. The only paper I found worthwhile was one read by this wonderfully eccentric physician. One of my neurosurgical colleagues insisted that he was a Shakespearean actor who had been hired to see whether he could fool the audience.

Intrigued, I called Skyrme and asked to meet with him. When I went up to his penthouse apartment, I found that he had eight magnums of champagne for our one-hour planned discussion. We wound up spending two hours and went out to lunch together afterward. One of the funniest things that happened was that I asked him how old he was, and when he told me, his wife, Margie, looked at him and said, "Are you really, dear?" This made me wonder about the Shakespearean actor.

When he came to La Crosse, Wisconsin, in May 1973 to demonstrate the rhyzolysis procedure to me, he made great fun of the fact that I was doing it in an operating room. He turned to his wife and said, "Imagine that, Margie, a proper operating room."

I asked him where he did his procedures and he said, "Oh, in the bloke's bed, on the floor, anywhere I can get them to lie still."

He continued his witty remarks right through my first rhyzolysis, as he called it. He refused to perform the procedure under my license; and as I stood poised with knife in hand, I fully expected him to jump up, click his heels, and exclaim, as I entered the patient's back, "You fool, there is no such procedure."

The patient, a thirty-year-old ranch wife, had been declared hysterical by a neurosurgeon. Following the simple procedure, her hysterical pain and numbness disappeared miraculously and remained gone the ten subsequent years that I knew her. Today, with proper prior

diagnostic facet nerve blocks, 70% of patients on whom I
perform a procedure, now done only with a needle and a
few drops of alcohol, are permanently, miraculously re-
lieved of pain for which conventional medicine has no
answer.

When I visited Skyrme in 1981, he used mer-
curochrome to cleanse a spot about the size of a thumbnail
before inserting the tenotomy blade into the spine. He
then used a sanitary napkin for a dressing. I asked him
why, and he said because it's inexpensive, easily available,
and holds a lot of blood.

Those are just a few of the extraordinary memories
that I have of Skyrme. I think Skyrme was one of those
wonderful eccentrics who intuitively perceived a great
solution for many people with chronic spinal pain.

Any approach that corrects misalignment of the spine
or reduces muscle spasm may relieve the physiological
pathology and lead to healing. There really is a scientific
law underlying each of these approaches. The miraculous
healings and insights provided by body therapy are none-
theless remarkable, for drugs and surgery cannot accomplish these benefits. As with all alternatives, a
comprehensive, holistic approach offers the best of all
worlds. The role of the allopath or osteopath is to evaluate
potentially serious illnesses. When there is no life-threatening problem, then ideally, postural, musculoskeletal
evaluation may yield a therapeutic breakthrough. Here, as
in all of medicine, intuition on the part of therapist and

client or patient is the only way to choose how far to go and which direction is safest and most effective.

Although I've not described Reichian therapy, Trager therapy, or a number of other body approaches, any one of them may provide the key for physical or emotional recovery. If significant relief is not initiated with from five to ten sessions of any such approach, then it is wise to look further in the vast warehouse of alternatives.

Facet denervation is another technique that defies many of the laws of conventional neurosurgery. This technique, which I learned from Skyrme Rees, is simple, safe, and, when done after two successful temporary blocks with a local anesthetic, effective in 80% of patients with migraine. The facet joints are the small joints on the back of the spine that overlap like shingles on a roof and allow us to move in many directions of twisting and turning. Current opinions in anatomy and physiology postulate that migraine is the result of a biochemical metabolic disorder. According to allopathic theory, there is no physical way in which a facet joint at C5-6 or 6-7 could cause a migraine. And, although usually the C2-3 facet is the problem in those migraine patients who benefit from facet denervation, occasionally I have seen miraculous results from denervating lower cervical points. Even at C2-3, the facets pose a challenge to the conventional attitude about migraine. Nevertheless, in a patient with frequent migraine and tender facets, especially at C2-3, a diagnostic nerve block with a local anesthetic may encourage our intuition to proceed. If on two occasions, such blocks totally relieve a migraine headache, then there is an 80% chance that facet denervation may help permanently. If a patient is still free of pain a week later, he or she has a 90% chance of permanent relief.

Despite conventional orthopedic and neurosurgical preoccupation with ruptured discs, it is my experience that a huge majority of patients with low back pain and even sciatica have mechanical problems with the facets. Hundreds of grateful patients have experienced the miracle of facet denervation.

I have followed many back-pain patients as long as fifteen years, and learned that if they received an initially good result from this safe procedure, they had a 90% chance of lasting pain relief with no side effects. This procedure is the extreme, perhaps, of alternative body therapies, but it is safe and worth serious consideration in many cases of spinal pain.

NOTE

1. *The Collected Papers of Irvin M. Korr,* ed. B. Peterson (Newark, OH: American Academy of Osteopathy, 1979).

Chapter 7

Nutrition

One of the most striking characteristics
of the modern treatment of disease is the return
to what used to be called the natural methods—
dieting, exercise, bathing and massage.
—Sir William Osler

As recently as 1910, beri beri, pellagra, and scurvy rav-
aged many lives. These diseases, which had never been
medically treatable, were essentially abolished with the
discovery of vitamins B1, B2, and C. The serious neurological illness, Wernicke's encephalopathy, which occasionally affects alcoholics, can be corrected almost instantly
with intravenous B vitamins. Partial paralysis from B12
deficiency may clear rapidly with administration of the
missing vitamin. Prior to the discovery of vitamins, these
illnesses were mysterious, and treatment was unavailing.
In the early days of vitamin therapy, such cures seemed
miraculous, even though they represented the simple
application of "laws" previously unknown.

For decades, those interested in nutrition have been ridiculed by the medical establishment, which even today teaches medical students only the most minimal information about nutrition. The public intuitively senses that something is wrong with this rigid conventional view.

As early as the 1940s, Dr. Weston A. Price of the Price/Pottenger Foundation demonstrated that many degenerative diseases result from poor diet.[1] Ironically, the poor diet in question is caused not by poverty but by the foods of prosperity—refined flour and white sugar—which deprive us of the natural vitamins and minerals of whole grains and natural sweeteners.

PURE DRINKING WATER

For example, it appears that dental caries—better known as tooth decay—is strongly linked to eating refined sugars. Yet we have treated it as a problem stemming from fluoride "deficiency," so we have added fluoride to the water supply of countless cities. Although fluoride assists in the prevention of dental caries, that fact does not prove a link between dental caries and fluoride deficiency. Excess fluoride may, in fact, be devastating to some people.

My own experience provides an example of fluoride's harmful effects. Although Dr. Fred Barge's literature provided me with evidence that drinking fluoridated water was unwise, when I underwent a cervical fusion for degenerative disc disease in 1967 I took large doses of fluoride (10 mg/day) for six weeks. About a year earlier, fluoride had been reported to assist in recalcification of bone in osteoporotic bones. I reasoned that fluoride would speed up the healing of my fusion. And indeed it did, but with the painful side effect of severe bursitis in my shoulders and hips.

It was not until some years later that I recognized fluoride as the cause of my bursitis. I had been giving my patients fluoride to help their fusions heal more rapidly, but they began developing bursitis at an alarming rate. Seeing a possible connection, I wrote the authors of the old osteoporotic article with my observation about bursitis and received the reply, "Yes, about 25% of patients given fluoride develop bursitis." A huge price to pay! But I am unaware of any scientific publication that warns people of this complication.

Scientific principles state that if a substance is toxic when taken in large doses on a short-term basis, it will also eventually prove toxic if taken in smaller doses over a longer period. (Of course, homeopathic remedies, which are diluted up to millions of times, are quite safe, and in treating allergies, tiny doses lead to desensitization.) Thus 10 mg. of fluoride daily over forty-two days is equal to approximately a year and a half of drinking fluoridated city water. Readers beware! When one drinks fluoridated water for twenty to eighty years, the total amount of fluoride consumed is formidable.

Nor do I consider chlorine a safe additive to our water supply. Recent studies conclude that men who drink just the recommended daily intake of city water, which is now chlorinated everywhere, have an increased incidence of bladder cancer. Of course, we cannot be sure whether the problem is the chlorine, the fluoride, or the combination of the two chemicals. I have also seen some evidence in my own practice that chlorine (and not sodium) is harmful to patients suffering from hypertension.[2] Furthermore, city water tastes awful, like drinking the water of a swimming pool. My advice is to avoid city water whenever possible.

I consider artificially softened water no better; it is loaded with sodium and chlorine. The simplest alternative for those who don't have a safe source of natural water is to invest in a good filter. Aqua King and Rexall offer inexpensive filters that can provide water that tastes as good as pure spring water, with virtually all fluoride and chlorine removed. They are available from Self-Health Systems.

Adding fluoride and chlorine to our drinking water is an example of what might be called "reverse miracles": serious complications that result from the failure of science to look adequately at known laws!

For those who have private wells, I recommend having your water tested at least once every five years for chemicals and bacteria. Get in touch with Water Test Corporation, 28 Daniel Plummer Road, Goffstown, NH 03045. Their phone number is (800) H2O-TEST.

JUNK FOODS

The use of white flour is another such problem. Enriched white flour is an oxymoron. It is highly deficient and totally incapable of sustaining life, whereas whole grain bread is the staff of life. White flour is deficient in virtually every natural nutrient—most particularly fiber, selenium, vitamin E, and vitamin B6. Cancer of the colon and diabetes, as well as dental caries and heart attack, are much more common in people who eat white flour to the exclusion of whole grains. White bread is anything but wholesome. Indeed, I consider almost all bread commercially available in the United States to be junk food. Even "whole wheat" bread is often half or more white flour and almost always loaded with chemical additives.

Find a bakery or health-food store that offers fresh whole-grain bread. It tastes better and is better for you. You can also bake bread at home, using natural ingredients and whole-grain flours. The process is easy, fun, and—if you knead the bread yourself—pleasantly therapeutic. And the bread will taste better than any manufactured loaf.

A second great culprit is refined sweeteners: white sugar, corn syrup, and fructose, among others. Americans consume their body weight in sugar *each year*. The resultant nutritional deficits are enormous. You cannot metabolize sugar without all the B vitamins and such minerals as zinc, chromium, and magnesium. Once again we contribute to significant degenerative diseases such as colon cancer, diabetes, heart disease, and dental caries by ignoring important scientific laws. Dr. Dennis Burkitt, a generation after Price and Pottenger, again has convincingly proven the lack of wisdom in continuing to use white sugar.[3]

Sugar's trigger of excess insulin release may be its

greatest attack upon the body. Anything that stimulates insulin excessively interferes with one of the body's most critical hormones: DHEA, or dehydroepiandrosterone. In our society at least, there is a steady decline in DHEA after the early twenties. This decline is highly correlated with every known illness, immune incompetence, and premature death.[4] (It would be most fascinating to study the DHEA levels in aborigines at age eighty!)

The carbonated soft drink is perhaps the single greatest contributor to the junk food craze. It is loaded, not only with sugar–about ten teaspoons per twelve ounces–but also with phosphorus, and often caffeine, as well as many non-natural chemicals. Every week the average American consumes more than a hundred teaspoons of sugar just from soft drinks.[5] Twenty teaspoons is the amount used in a glucose tolerance test, enough to trigger a massive insulin release.

Moreover, phosphorus interferes with absorption of calcium and magnesium, thus further straining our nutritional resources. There is simply nothing good to be said for soda pop or phosphate of soda. If you can't avoid soda entirely, at least drink as little as you can.

Diet sodas are no improvement over sugary sodas. No artificial sweeteners are good for you, or essential to nutrition. In one sense, they are junk food, for they are not natural or real. And aspartame is particularly harmful for some people, causing headaches, anxiety, agitation, high blood pressure, and seizures.

CAFFEINE AND ALCOHOL

Another problem of soda may be its caffeine content, although that issue is debatable. The human body has no need for caffeine, but there is equally no convincing evidence of harm from moderate caffeine intake. Moderation means two cups of coffee or three of tea daily. You should drink less of colas, for they have junk food additives. Even with decaffeinated coffee, huge quantities may not be optimal. Cocoa, mate tea, and gota kola also contain caffeine.

On the other hand, excess caffeine is a tremendous aggravator of headaches, especially migraine. Taken after 3 P.M., caffeine interferes with Stage Four sleep, the sleep necessary for restoration as well as DHEA and beta endorphin replenishment. I strongly suspect that even decaffeinated coffee taken after 3 P.M. is harmful to good sleep.

Alcohol, like caffeine, is devoid of nutritional value, yet it may not be entirely bad for you. Although they share virtually nothing else in their religions, neither the Mormons nor the Seventh-Day Adventists drink alcohol, and these two groups have roughly half the incidence of cancer as average Americans—and both groups live longer.[6] The major factor appears to be their avoidance of alcohol and tobacco. It is difficult to separate the two factors.

On the other hand, it appears that alcohol, in moderation, may not be particularly harmful. Moderation is generally defined as a maximum of one and a half ounces of whiskey or its equivalent per day. The equivalent is about six ounces of wine and twelve to eighteen ounces of beer. In an individual who is otherwise healthy and living a good lifestyle, drinking in moderation may be relatively neutral. I would remind you, however, that alcohol is not needed; it does cause excess insulin release, similar to sugar; deprives you of essential vitamins and minerals, especially magnesium, which is generally deficient in our diets; and it may aggravate DHEA depletion. The best advice is to avoid or at least minimize alcohol, as it is highly addicting to some individuals.

ARTIFICIALLY HYDROGENATED FATS

Another great offender is artificially hydrogenated fat, which converts essential cis-linoleic acid into dangerous trans-linoleic acid, which is at least as bad for you as beef fat and worse than pork fat. Margarine and all the solid vegetable shortenings deplete the foundation for prostaglandin E1, one of the natural health promoters and immune enhancers.

Most commercial peanut butters are loaded with artificially hydrogenated fat and added sugar. Choose instead old-fashioned peanut butter for a spread. Use butter, olive oil, or canola oil for cooking.

Some of the non-fat dairy products taste almost as good as dairy and are free of the artificially hydrogenated plaque. Non-fat sour cream is excellent. Avoid the cream substitutes too, both the powdered and the liquid; I consider them to be filled with pure junk.

WHAT TO AVOID: A BRIEF GUIDE

If I were to list all the junk food filling our grocery shelves, it would fill a book twice the size of this one. Read labels and reject all pseudofood products with the words:

white (except fish!)

artificial

hardened

hydrogenated

partially

substitute

sugar

corn sweetener/syrup

enriched

additives

conditioner

processed

bleached

flavored

Beyond these chemically altered products, today's food is riddled with pesticides, herbicides, antibiotics, and hormones picked up at various stages of the food chain. None of these is safe or health-promoting. Even milk is so altered as to be far less nourishing than it was fifty years ago. Although pasteurization is vital to avoid some poten-

tial infectious diseases, homogenization is at best useless
and at worst harmful. There is evidence that homogenization alters milk fat in such a way that it increases the risk
of atherosclerosis.[7] Moreover, milk cows are now being
dosed with artificial bovine growth hormone. Some milk
(as well as other foods) is then processed with radiation,
and thus denaturalized.

CHOOSING A HEALTHY DIET

In general it is, however, useless for the average person to
worry excessively about aspects of nutrition that we can't
change easily. The best you can do is to eat a wide variety
of real food, as near natural as possible. There is no
evidence that beef or pork in moderation is harmful. In
moderation means one to two servings per week of lean,
non-fried meat. Fish, chicken (non-fried and without the
skin), and turkey (without skin) are relatively good. But a
maximum of eight ounces of flesh food per day is quite
adequate. Beyond meat, eat as many servings as desired of
fresh vegetables and fruits, raw or steamed. Include some
nuts and seeds and a generous amount of whole grains,
such as oatmeal, 100% whole wheat, and brown rice. And
don't forget dried legumes. They're as good a source of
protein as beef, and a lot cheaper.

Enjoy eggs, one or two per day, non-fried, as long as
you don't have familial hypercholesterolemia. Remember that ten minutes of stress leads your body to produce
more cholesterol than you get from an egg![8]

Learn to season with herbs, especially coriander, cumin, and turmeric, which give vegetables a heartier flavor. Almost all herbs and spices are healthful and enjoyable.

Among the vast array of unusual diets, there is some evidence that the Gerson diet, the macrobiotic diet, and the Anopson raw-food diet help some patients who have cancer.[9] But if you eat real foods and are not seriously ill, such diets are of no particular value. My personal dietary recommendation to those with serious immune deficiency illnesses, such as cancer, AIDS, lupus, rheumatoid arthritis, and advanced psoriasis is given in Chapter 10. So is nutritional advice for those who have high cholesterol.

Finally, in our polluted, fast-paced society, unless you live on an organic farm, raise most of your food, and travel minimally, I recommend some nutritional insurance. The evidence is excellent that megavitamins, within the limits to be outlined, are good for you. A study carried out in 1994 and widely touted was seriously flawed: in Scandinavia, smokers were given rather modest doses of vitamin C, beta carotene, and vitamin E without a decreased incidence of lung cancer.[10] The dosages used were less than I recommend for those with a healthy lifestyle, let alone those with the most unhealthy of all habits, smoking.

Consider the following recommendations:

- Beta Carotene, 25,000 units daily. I recommend that everybody take some—up to 200,000

units per day for people who have immune
system problems or allergies and even healthy
people–a minimum of one capsule containing
25,000 units per day for maintenance.

- Life Support, an excellent complete multivitamin, multimineral supplement, 3 a day; or Life
Extension Mix, the most comprehensive multivitamin, multimineral supplement, 9 a day.

- Vitamin C, at least two grams a day (beyond
that in the multivitamin mixtures).

EAT REAL FOOD

Real food may enhance good health and is always better
than junk food. The miracle of nutrition ultimately comes
from avoiding the squalid swamp of artificial, processed
junk foods. My advice is to avoid refined foods, artificial
sweeteners, artificially hydrogenated fats, and any future
manufactured pseudofood. Eat right and expect a miracle!

NOTES

1. Weston A. Price, *Nutrition and Physical Degeneration*
   (Santa Monica, CA: The Price-Pottenger Nutrition
   Foundation, 1945).

2. Dr. Dean Burke, *The Oakland (California) Tribune*
   (June 22, 1975), p. 12.

3. D.P. Burkitt, M.D., and H.D. Trolwell, M.D., eds.,
   Refined Carbohydrate Foods and Disease: Some Implica-

tions of Dietary Fiber (New York: Academic Press, 1975).

4. S.M. Haffner, R.A.Valdez, L. Mykanen, M.P. Stern, and M.S. Katz, "Decreased Testosterone and Dehydroepiandrosterone Sulfate Concentrations Are Associated with Increased Insulin and Glucose Concentrations in Nondiabetic Men," *Metabolism* 43 (May 1994): 599–603; A.G. Schwartz and L.L. Pasko, "Cancer Chemoprevention with the Adrenocortical Steroid Dehydroepiandrosterone and Structural Analogs," *Journal of Cell Biochemistry,* Supplement 17G (1992): 73–70; F. Stahl, D. Schnorr, C. Pilz, G. Dorner, "Dehydroepiandrosterone Levels in Patients with Prostatic Cancer, Heart Diseases and Under Surgery Stress," *Experiments in Clinical Endocrinology* 99 (1992): 68–70.

5. "Too Much Sugar," *Consumer Reports* 43 (March 1978): 136–142.

6. Roland L. Phillips, "Cancer among Seventh-Day Adventists," *Journal of Environmental Pathology and Toxicology* 3(1980): 157–169; Roland L. Phillips, Jan W. Kuzma, and Terry M. Lotz, "Cancer Mortality among Comparable Members versus Nonmembers of the Seventh-Day Adventist Church," in *Banbury Report 4: Cancer Incidence in Defined Populations,* (1980) : 93–108.

7. Gershon Hepner, Richard Fried, Sachiko St. Jeor, Lydia Fusetti, and Robert Morin, "Hypercholes-

terolemic Effect of Yogurt and Milk, 1–3," *American Journal of Clinical Nutrition* 32 (January 1979): 19–24.

8. D.F. Horobin, "A New Concept of Lifestyle-Related Cardiovascular Disease: The Importance of Interactions between Cholesterol, Essential Fatty Acids, Prostaglandin E1 and Thromboxane A2," *Medical Hypotheses* 6 (1980): 785–800.

9. Severin L. Schaeffer, *Instinctive Nutrition* (Berkeley, CA: Celestial Arts, 1987); Michio Kushi, *The Book of Macrobiotics: The Universal Way of Health and Happiness* (New York: Harper and Row, 1978); Max Gerson, *A Cancer Therapy* (Del Mar, CA: Totality Books, 1958).

10. The Alpha Tocopherol, Beta Carotene Cancer Prevention Study Group, "The Effect of Vitamin E and Beta Carotene on the Incidence of Lung Cancer and Other Cancers in Male Smokers," *New England Journal of Medicine* 330 (April 14, 1994): 1029–35.

PART TWO

Creating Your Own Miracles

Chapter 8

Conventional vs. Alternative Medicine

Faith in us,
faith in our drugs and methods,
is the great stock in trade
of the profession.
—Sir William Osler

Traditional medicine is the kind that has been used for more than a hundred years. *Conventional* medicine is the medical practice that is currently in vogue among the majority of M.D.s and D.O.s. The major advantages of the latter are tremendous technological advances in diagnosis and surgery, along with moderate advances in pharmacology. For treatment of significant acute illnesses, conventional medicine is virtually the only reasonable choice.

137

Some symptoms that indicate immediate conventional medical attention is needed are:

- Sudden acute pain, especially of head, chest, or abdomen
- Paralysis or numbness, partial or total, in any area of the body
- Loss of consciousness
- Seizures
- Fever above 101°F
- Difficulty in breathing
- Confusion or significant personality changes
- Diastolic blood pressure above 100
- Irregular or very rapid heartbeat, or sudden drop in heart rate below fifty beats per minute
- Significant swelling or redness of any part of the body
- Inability to urinate or defecate
- Bleeding from wounds or unknown causes
- Rapid weight loss, frequent urination, and excessive thirst
- Any of the seven warning signs of cancer: a sore that won't heal; any change in a wart or mole; indigestion more than occasionally or problems with swallowing; change in bowel or

bladder habits; a persistent cough or hoarse-
ness; a lump in the breast or elsewhere; any
unusual bleeding or discharge

It's also appropriate to consult medical or surgical specialists for the following problems:

- Any life-threatening illness
- Psychosis
- Severe dementia
- Cognitive problems, which require at least a
  CT scan and neuropsychological testing
- Fractures
- Worrisome illnesses with uncertainty as to
  diagnosis
- Heart attacks
- Acute stroke
- Coma
- Acute paralysis
- Meningitis, encephalitis
- Glomerulonephritis
- Rheumatic fever
- Cancer
- Ruptured intervertebral disc with significant
  neurologic deficit

- Severe degenerative disease of the hip
- Diabetes
- Tuberculosis
- Diarrhea in infants
- Other diseases in infants
- Vaccinations*
- Pregnancy
- Whenever in doubt

Until we have widely available techniques for natural restoration of DHEA, I believe that all patients with these illnesses or conditions should have their DHEA measured and be treated with DHEA and the Ring of Fire. I suspect many lives could be saved and the quality of the patient's remaining life greatly improved through this practice.

Many infections, especially bacterial ones, can be treated relatively safely and promptly with antibiotics. In viral infections, alternative medicine is often superior, as it is most often in chronic illnesses. Innumerable alternative medical approaches are available; to discuss all of them would require an encyclopedia. I will here discuss some of the treatments I have found to be most effective, especially those that have been associated with apparent miracles, where conventional medicine has little to offer. They are listed in order of relative importance.

---

* Despite the concern of some individuals, I believe conventional medicine's greatest advance has been vaccinations.

SELF-HYPNOSIS AND BIOFEEDBACK

At least 80% of chronic illnesses can be markedly improved with these time-honored approaches, which are foolishly ignored by conventional physicians. As early as 1969, more than 2600 scientific papers proved the efficacy of autogenic training, a form of self-hypnosis. The addition of biofeedback in 1971 made autogenic training scientifically understandable, but for the subsequent quarter century it remained almost unknown and largely unused. Many of the miraculous healings I've reported are the result of using Biogenics, my organized form of biofeedback and self-hypnosis. I believe that acupuncture and Biogenics should be the first considerations in most problems not safely treatable by conventional medicine. Biogenics is described in detail in my book, *The Self-Healing Workbook* (Element Books, 1993), available at many bookstores. For audiotapes of the major exercises, contact Self-Health Systems.

ACUPUNCTURE

Acupuncture, when performed by a well-trained acupuncturist, is effective for treatment of many types of pain. It is also useful to treat severe anxiety and PMS. It can provide symptomatic improvement of many chronic illnesses, and it restores fertility in two-thirds of infertile men. This latter accomplishment alone establishes acupuncture as a miraculous treatment, since conventional medicine can't compete!

TRANSCUTANEOUS ELECTRICAL NERVE STIMULATION

For pain, acute or chronic, Transcutaneous Electrical Nerve Stimulation (TENS) vies with acupuncture in efficacy. Any physician unfamiliar with TENS is ignorant. If your physician knows nothing about TENS and fails to recommend it, find one who does. Although widely available, it is used less than 5% of the time when symptoms indicate its appropriateness. Almost totally safe, TENS should be considered at least as an adjunct in every type of pain.

CRANIAL ELECTRICAL STIMULATION

Cranial electrical stimulation (CES), which is a safe and effective treatment for depression, insomnia, and jet lag, may help relieve pain as well. It boosts beta endorphins, the natural feel-good narcotics, and serotonin, an essential balancing neurochemical. I consider CES the treatment of choice for depression and insomnia, for most facial and head pains, and any pain that is hyperesthetic, where light touch is felt as pain.

PHOTOSTIMULATION

Photostimulation is the most useful adjunct for relaxation, and the use of the Relaxation Response is effective in 80% of chronic illnesses. If you have trouble relaxing enough to do deep relaxation for health maintenance or to fall asleep, I recommend the Shealy RelaxMate. The RelaxMate is a pair of goggles with small flashing lights in front of each eye. These lights can be adjusted to flicker from 1 to 7.5 cycles per second, the frequencies associated with the deepest states of relaxation. At least 90% of people who use it feel deeply relaxed within ten minutes.

BODY THERAPY

A wide variety of body therapies makes choosing a treatment for various problems somewhat difficult. For spinal pain, manipulation by a trained osteopathic physician (D.O.) or a competent chiropractor (D.C.) is certainly to be considered. There is some risk if movement is too vigorous in the neck or when used on patients who have osteoporosis or metastatic cancer.

Postural correction is helpful to most people who are in pain. The correction may be done through Alexander therapy, Lennon exercises, Rolfing, or Feldenkrais therapy. These techniques are not widely practiced, so private consultation may be needed to help you decide on one of these approaches. Some physical therapists apply several techniques to assist in development of good posture.

Massage of any type may help reduce muscle tension or spasms, assist relaxation, increase circulation, and just feel good.

Trager therapy is another form of body-mind alignment that may be helpful to people with tension/postural problems. It consists of a passive, gentle movement of head, shoulders, neck, and legs.

HOMEOPATHY

The principle of homeopathy, which is based on the law
of similars, is closer to the desensitization concept in
allergy treatment than to anything else in medicine. The
theory behind homeopathy is essentially as follows: If a
measurable dose of any chemical can produce a specific
symptom, then diluting that dose thousands or millions of
times may produce a product that treats the symptom. The
most obvious example is allergy to bee stings. If you dilute
the venom adequately, repeated doses may render you
insensitive or immune to bee venom. These microdoses
are below the threshold of tolerance, so they do not prove
poisonous.

Long rejected by conventional medicine, homeopathy benefits many people with immune and autoimmune
disorders. The greatest single miracle I've seen with homeopathy is reversal of scleroderma, a connective-tissue
disease usually fatal and untreatable by conventional
medicine.

Patients with rheumatoid arthritis may also benefit
from this safe alternative. It stands head and shoulders
above prednisone, gold shots, and methotrexate. Homeopathy is best used without drugs and combined with
Biogenics for rheumatoid arthritis. The rheumatoid arthritis preparation from Beaumont Labs is the one I recommend.

The homeopathic preparation called cocculus may
provide rapid, miraculous relief from vertigo, a severe

manifestation of dizziness. Conventional medicine's drug approach is mediocre at best, and what it offers involves significant undesirable side effects: dry mouth, confusion, even brain damage with spontaneous tremors.

In influenza, for which allopathy (conventional medicine) has no primary treatment, homeopathic oscillococcinum may provide remarkable relief. These homeopathic preparations are available at many health-food stores.

GigaTENS

If it were available in the United States now, GigaTENS would be my Number One choice for alternative treatment. I hope that by the time this book is published, GigaTENS will be available in the US. A 5-10-K application has been filed with the FDA, which should lead to availability by late 1995. At this time, somewhat similar equipment is available only in the Ukraine, where more than 200,000 patients have already been treated with it. On my trip to the Ukraine, the researchers reported that its success rate ranges from 50% of patients with narcotic addiction to 85% of those with rheumatoid arthritis. Our preliminary results at the Shealy Institute in some seventy-five patients suggest that this is the most important innovation in medical history. Keep alert for its introduction. Undoubtedly a national press release will be disseminated when the device is available.

GigaTENS is a battery-powered electrical device that

puts out a billionth of a watt at the rate of fifty-two to seventy-eight billion cycles per second. This is almost solar homeopathy, but in contrast to what is possible in homeopathy, the output of GigaTENS is measurable with oscilloscopes. Nuclear physicists in the Ukraine told my colleague, Saul Liss, and me that human DNA vibrates at from fifty-two to seventy-eight billion cycles per second, so what GigaTENS does is essentially to recharge the human electrical battery.

DEHYDROEPIANDROSTERONE

Dehydroepiandrosterone (DHEA) is the single most important chemical in the human body. It is the blueprint hormone produced in the adrenal glands and reflective of life reserves. The only lab I trust for administering this test is Corning-Nichols in Capistrano, California. Fortunately, its services are available by mail throughout the United States. Any other reference labs I know of are unreliable for this test, and I do not recommend using them.

Optimal levels of DHEA for men are 750 to 1250 ng/dL, 550 to 980 in women. When the levels fall below 180 in men and 130 in women, supplementation with DHEA is essential. It does require a prescription. We recommend Thayer's Colonial Pharmacy, 1101 East Colonial Drive, Orlando, FL, 32803, 1-800-848-4809, for the timed-release capsule. Adding from 50 to 100 mg/day for men and 20 to 75 mg. for women may be adequate and safe. There is some evidence that natural progesterone cream (available from Self-Health Systems) will increase DHEA levels significantly, and it may be worthwhile to try that before deciding to take DHEA orally. Early results with GigaTENS demonstrate that it, too, will raise DHEA. If so, GigaTENS will become the first choice for virtually all chronic illnesses and an adjunct in acute ones.

NUTRITION

Although good nutrition is essential for health maintenance and may assist in restoration of health for most patients, it is difficult to prove cures with improvement in nutrition. The diet of choice for most individuals is a wide variety of real food, avoiding as much as possible the processed foods, sugar, soda, white bread, and hydrogenated fats. Up to two cups of coffee or tea, before 5 P.M., is acceptable. You should drink two quarts per day of real water, bottled or filtered.

I recommend this preventive program of nutritional supplements (available from Self-Health Systems):

1 tablet daily of VitaMin 100 (W)

2 grams vitamin C (timed release)

25,000 units beta carotene

2 tabs Pycnogenol per day

6 to 9 grams per day of borage or black currant seed oil

For those with allergies or immune deficiency, add the following:

> Beta carotene, a total of 200,000 units per day
>
> Vitamin C, up to a total of 10 grams per day, if needed
>
> 1 gram calcium each morning
>
> 2 capsules, 125 mg. each, of magnesium taurate at bedtime
>
> And don't forget DHEA and your Ring of Fire!

All these products are vegetarian.

Herbs

For post-menopausal women, I recommend adding to the above list three tablets of Herb-F every day. For men over 50, I would add the same dosage of Herb-M, and if it doesn't add zest to your sex life, switch to Yohimbe. For prostate enlargement or symptoms, I would add three tablets of Super Saw Palmetto per day. All these supplements are available from Self-Health Systems.

For more information on herbs, consult Maria Treben's book, *Health Through God's Pharmacy*.

SPIRITUAL HEALING

Prayer and spiritual healing are worth serious consideration in every illness. Occasionally, grace results in miraculous healing. And as Olga Worrall says, "Another touch of healing never hurt anyone."

Some healing sources are:

Ron Roth, PO Box 1064, La Salle, IL 60301

Miatek Wirkus, 4803 St. Elmo Avenue, Bethesda, MD 20814

New Life Clinic, Thursday mornings, Mt. Washington United Methodist Church, Baltimore, MD.

INTUITIVE DIAGNOSIS

Sometimes, if you are totally frustrated by the failure of conventional or alternative medicine to come up with a satisfactory diagnosis or prescription, a talented intuitive diagnostician may be of help. Most often in such situations, the problem is one of unresolved psychospiritual stress. Nevertheless, if you contact a reputable medical intuitive, you may receive insight to assist you in your healing journey. Contact Self-Health Systems for a referral to those we believe to be honest and talented in this field.

PAST LIFE THERAPY

In a few situations, insight is blocked. Past life therapy may help you when all else fails. Contact Self-Health Systems for a referral.

INSIGHT MEDITATION CHAMBER

In general, I believe personal insight is the most effective tool for moving beyond blocks. I have created a simple plan for building an insight meditation chamber, which is inexpensive and a great way to create a sacred space. (See Chapter 9.)

MUSIC BEDS

For optimal deep relaxation and insight assistance, a vibrating music bed is unbeatable. Commercial units cost from $4,500 to $45,000, but for $200 you can build one using your own hi-fi equipment. (See Chapter 9.)

LIGHT

As a general contributor to health, natural light is one of the great benefits ignored by conventional medicine. Ideally, you should be outside without any glasses for two hours or more per day. The best times are before noon and after 2 P.M. Even being in the shade is beneficial. Light and the natural solar giga frequencies help regulate the pineal gland and thus the pituitary gland and all hormones. For prevention of osteoporosis and breast cancer, nothing is more powerful. There is some evidence that adequate full-spectrum light may assist in seasonal affective disorder (winter depression), PMS, alcoholism, drug addiction, multiple sclerosis, Alzheimer's syndrome, colon and rectal cancer, panic attacks, rheumatoid arthritis, infertility, hyperactivity in children, chronic fatigue syndrome, and even dental caries. You can't afford to live in a cave![1]

If your job prevents you from being outside, you should use full-spectrum fluorescents (available from Self-Health Systems) in your work area; be outside four or more hours on weekend days and consider installing at least four full-spectrum lights as close as possible to your indoor exercise area. If you must wear glasses outside, get full-spectrum plastic lenses. In summer, especially from 10 A.M. to 2 P.M. or when outside with snow on the ground, you should wear sunglasses. Obviously, you always avoid looking directly at the sun.

PSYCHONEUROIMMUNOLOGY AND STRESS

Just as the head bone is ultimately connected to the toe bones, the brain/mind is connected with everything else. In contrast to the common medical belief that body and mind are separate entities, your brain/mind is the key to health and your most important "alternative" healer. For almost two decades now, science has reaffirmed the age-old wisdom that you are what you think—or, as Edgar Cayce put it, "Mind is the Builder." Two totally separate fields have proved this connection: biofeedback and psychoneuroimmunology.

Just as Edmond Jacobsen demonstrated in 1929 and J.H. Schultz in 1932 that every physiological function is improved by deep relaxation and autogenic training, biofeedback has now proved that with proper training, every function that can be measured can be controlled. Biofeedback provides the faith by proving that your thinking or visualizing actually *changes* bodily functions.

Thus it speeds up the learning process. For headache and blood-pressure control, for management of reflex sympathetic dystrophy, for treatment of attention deficit disorder, and even for epilepsy, biofeedback helps the brain/mind focus and learn.

During the past fifteen years, the new science of psychoneuroimmunology has demonstrated that every thought is even more, perhaps, than a prayer, as so eloquently proposed by Ambrose Worrall. Every thought, properly focused, may be the answer to your prayers!

Many marvelous books have touched on this subject. Among my favorites are: *Mind as Healer, Mind as Slayer,* by Kenneth Pelletier (Delacorte Press, 1977); *Who Gets Sick,* by Blair Justice (Peak Press, 1987); and *Minding the Body, Mending the Mind,* by Joan Borysenko (Addison-Wesley, 1987). These books explore the most elegant science of all time, proving that thinking, imagining, and feeling are the control mechanisms for the hypothalamus, the autonomic nervous system, and the immune system. Most studies in psychoneuroimmunology focus upon the impact of mental or emotional changes on lymphocytes and immune globulins—major aspects of immune function. The immune system ultimately is the most pervasive, inclusive, and representative of total body functions. There are more illnesses involving the immune system than all other systems combined.

Candace Pert, one of the leaders in the field of psychoneuroimmunology and the study of the various neurochemicals involved with attitude and emotions, has explained that scientific revolutions happen in this way: "Most people deny them and resist them. And then there is more and more of an explosion, and there is a paradigm shift."[2] In her field we are not yet at the level of an explosion, for the vast majority of physicians, scientists, and lay persons do not accept or understand the tremendous research of the past decade and a half.

Hans Selye emphasizes that subliminal amounts of chemical stressors—that is, amounts below the threshold of stress—are additive. For example, it may take one whole cigarette to trigger an alarm reaction in an individual who has never been exposed to cigarettes before, or one whole cup of coffee to precipitate an alarm reaction, or one whole sugar-coated donut. Although one-third of each of these would not by itself trigger an alarm reaction, when one-third of each is taken together, the combination does trigger an alarm reaction. This is the nature of the subtle interactions of stress.

Just as we are subject to all of these interacting chemical stressors, we must also undergo interacting chemical, physical, emotional, and electromagnetic stressors. For example, workers who are exposed to very intense electromagnetic energy for eight hours a day on the job have increased incidences of brain cancer and leukemia. Yet not everyone in these jobs develops brain cancer or leukemia. Some day we may be able to study the subtle interactions of the people who have developed such illnesses in such environments and examine and measure their emotional stress, their chemical stress, and their

physical inactivity, all of which would contribute to the
total effect on the body. I want to emphasize here the
complexity and subtleness of the interactions that lead to
health or illness.

Many of the organisms that cause illness in our bodies
are clearly long-term residents–saprophytes, if you will.
Perhaps the easiest example to understand is the way we
are affected by the fever blister virus, *Herpes labialis.*
Apparently, most of us are infected with it in infancy.
Some people have fever blisters on their lips or nose quite
frequently. Some women break out with a fever blister
with every menstrual cycle. Other individuals develop the
blister under the least amount of extra stress. I had one
fever blister when I was a child and another in my teens,
and I had no other, no matter how many other intervening
stressors came along, until I was bitten by a brown recluse
spider near my left eye. I awoke in the morning with the
usual black necrotic area, my eye swollen shut, and a fever
blister. I have not had another one since–my resistance in
general is good. But many other individuals develop a
fever blister with any emotional crisis.

Dr. Stewart Wolf, a long-time clinical researcher in
medicine and physiology, who now works in Pennsylva-
nia, has suggested that "disease is a way of life."[3] One study
has shown that one-quarter of us experience more than
half of all illnesses and more than two-thirds of all the total
days of disability. Those who are more dissatisfied and
discontented with their lives had more illnesses. A survey
showed that among both men and women, those who

have the lowest morale and greatest job dissatisfaction always perceived themselves as having more stress; they are the people who turn out to have the most frequent illnesses.

A major study at Harvard Medical School by pediatricians Roger Meyer and Robert Haggerty, who followed sixteen families with a total of a hundred persons throughout a year, showed that streptococcal illnesses and other upper respiratory problems were four times more frequent after episodes in which the families felt that they had experienced a stressful experience. Families that underwent higher levels of ongoing chronic stress suffered significantly more streptococcal illnesses than those who did not.[4]

Another interesting study involved Native Americans who were forced out of their simple nomadic life to a "higher" standard of living on reservations; it showed that the change caused a marked increase in deaths from tuberculosis. To these people, being uprooted from the land of their forbears led them to a sense of hopelessness.[5] On the other hand, Portuguese men immigrating to Canada because they believed that they would have new jobs and a new future actually improved in health. The sense of loss of control is one of the most critical in the precipitation of disease, but moving itself is not a major stressor if one is happy about it.[6]

As early as 1910, Sir William Osler, the father of American medicine, declared that angina pectoris was a result of stress and strain. Whether stress produces difficulty, however, depends upon the way we view our trouble. If we have a sense of control and a feeling that a challenge is an opportunity, then positive peptides–little chains of amino acids that help us feel good and protect our immune system–are produced in the brain. Being open to change and feeling involved and part of the action can increase our resistance to illness, but a sense of helplessness depresses our immune system and decreases our resistance immensely.

The work of Suzanne Kobasa and her colleagues has been particularly important. She found that executives and managers who considered change to be good did well under extreme stress, and those who considered change to be bad did poorly. Obviously, those who have a sense of control and a commitment to being involved in life do better. Feeling in control gives people a sense of meaning, direction, and excitement. Kobasa considers a person's feeling of personal control, sense of commitment, and ability to accept challenge as the keys to "psychological hardiness."[7]

The most important key to control is the ability to look at a bad situation, analyze it, and see that there is a way to reduce the stress it brings into your life. In other words, if you look at losses, hurts, frustrations, and other stressors as challenges rather than as the results of victimization, you have better control. You can alter the events or the effects of the event so that they are less stressful. You cannot afford the luxury of being a pessimist.

There are many ways of coping with stress. These involve:

- acting to change the problem, if change is possible;
- viewing the problem as a challenge rather than an affront or an intentional hurt;
- getting adequate physical exercise;
- eating properly;
- and regularly engaging in deep relaxation.

Over and over again, psychoneuroimmunological studies show that lymphocytes and antibodies–which give us the ability to resist infection and cancer–are affected by our basic attitudes of happiness or positivity as opposed to sadness, depression, hopelessness, and pessimism. Our physiology, the chemistry and electricity of the human body, is constantly affected every moment of the day, not just by what we eat and drink and breathe but also by how we move and how we feel. Dr. Robert Good, another leader in the field of psychoneuroimmunology and former president and director of Memorial Sloan-Kettering Cancer Hospital in New York, has emphasized that a positive attitude and a constructive frame of mind all improve our ability to resist infections, allergies, and autoimmune disorders in cancer, whereas depression and pessimism decrease our ability to do so.[8]

It is almost an anti-miracle that so few people realize now that every major illness–cancer, heart disease, diabetes, hypertension, stroke–and most accidents are more the result of our attitudes than of all other measurable factors combined. Although many books can be written documenting these effects, it is perhaps wise to conclude this section with a brief reminder of the work of Dr. Heinz Isaac. In studying some 13,000 people followed over a period of some twenty years, he found that 75% of those people who died of cancer had a lifelong pattern of feeling hopeless; 15% had a lifelong pattern of being angry; and more than 9% had a lifelong pattern of mixtures of the first two. At the same time, 75% of those people who died of heart disease had a lifelong pattern of being angry; 15% had a lifelong pattern of feeling helpless; and more than 9% had a lifelong pattern of a mixture of those two.

Among smokers, those who have superb self-esteem and who feel that happiness is an inside job—who would be considered psychologically hearty by Kobasa or "self-actualized" by Abraham Maslow—all have a very low (0.8%) incidence of developing cancer. Non-smoking people of this type develop cancer only 0.3% of the time. But among smokers who have a lifelong pattern of hope-lessness, the incidence of developing cancer is 28%, or roughly a hundred times that of the non-smoking, well-adjusted person and thirty times that of the smoking well-adjusted person. Thus *an attitude of hopelessness or chronic depression has a thirty times greater negative effect upon health than does smoking itself,* which has only a 2.7 times negative effect upon health.[9] You can't afford the luxury of chronic anger, guilt, anxiety, or depression.

The hierarchy of psychoneuroimmunology looks something like this:

Your genes and early environment (for the first six years) are critical, but there are influences from the cosmos (electromagnetic waves and divine will).

These basic factors are influenced by your attitude, and attitudes strongly affect your electrical and chemical stability.

Attitude most directly affects the central limbic system, the "emotional" center of the brain. From this center come the strongest influences upon the pineal gland, hypothalamus, and pituitary gland—the Master Control System—for all hormones and neurochemicals, including the hormones that regulate sleep, mood, and comfort, as well as the regulators of parathyroid, thyroid, adrenals, and testicles or ovaries. Growth hormone, prolactin, and oxytocin (the nurturing hormone in both men and women) are more affected by moment-to-moment attitude than by any other factor.

The next level of response is in norepinephrine (adrenalin); serotonin (the sleep, depression, and migraine regulator); beta endorphins (the feel-good natural narcotic); and melatonin (a major regulator of sleep and an anti-aging hormone).

Cortisol, a powerful anti-inflammatory chemical, is released as a primary response to stress of all kinds. Increased cortisol depresses production of DHEA, the most important hormone in the body. DHEA regulates testosterone and estrogen production, and the DHEA level ultimately influences all the hormones in the body.

The usual blood chemistries (sodium, potassium, protein, cholesterol, and so on) are balanced when all the higher-level chemicals and hormones are optimal. Finally, the white blood cells, lymphocytes, and globulins (immune proteins) are the end-product reflectors of immune competence.

Psychoneuroimmunology often looks only at lymphocytes and globulins in relation to mood or attitude. But all the hormones and chemicals mentioned—and many more—are ultimately the result of this complex chemical reaction to attitude!

OTHER ALTERNATIVES

Innumerable other techniques are touted as being useful, but in most cases, I doubt that any of them is as good as those I've listed. Nevertheless, if you haven't achieved your goals and have really applied yourself to the techniques described above, then contact the American Holistic Medical Association or the American Holistic Nurses' Association (both at 4101 Lake Boone Trail, Suite 201, Raleigh, NC 27607) for lists of practitioners and further suggestions.

Medicine has evolved along with all other aspects of life. In the earliest days of humanity there were, undoubtedly, illnesses and accidents that rendered individuals incapable of functioning. The natural tendency of human beings to nurture led to trial-and-error treatments. Many undoubtedly died in the days of pre-science, when someone intuitively tried some unusual herb and learned that it was poisonous.

Primitive people even performed open surgery on the skull. Skeletal remains show that some persons miraculously survived such surgery; their skulls show clear-cut long-standing healing before these brave souls died. Bones were set, too, perhaps crudely.

Reasonably early in time, the use of rituals became a major method of healing. These shamanistic events appear to have been built largely on ceremonies designed to create faith, hope, or belief–the beginning of the placebo effect. Such tribal healers used herbs, laying on of hands, ritual dance, affirmations, incantations, and, above all, powerful commands.

Acupuncture was developed more than four thousand years ago. At least two thousand years ago music, relaxation, massage, aromatherapy, color therapy, and cognitive psychotherapy were available. Indeed, the father of all medicine, Aesculapius, used dream therapy to diagnose and treat patients in ancient Greece. Of course, none of the miracles of modern medicine then existed.

Most modern science is, in general, only about two hundred years old. Medical science as a whole is even younger. Before 1940, medical science offered minimal hope of cure. Medicine, like most fields, has not been kind to original thinkers. In fact, almost every innovator has been virtually martyred or, at best, ridiculed and attacked. William Harvey, credited with the discovery of circulation, was attacked viciously by his colleagues. Ignaz Phillip Semmelweis's discovery that physicians transmitted puerperal (childbed) fever was ridiculed and ignored, although thousands of women died painfully and needlessly because of the arrogant refusal of physicians to wash their hands! Puerperal fever was one of the first serious iatrogenic—physician-caused—diseases. Today hundreds of such diseases infect patients. Even twenty years ago a book of several hundred pages detailed the iatrogenic diseases that were prevalent. Today at least 25% of hospitalized patients suffer complications that should have been avoided.[10]

The safest and most effective treatment of any illness will always be prevention. Experts estimate that 85% of all illnesses are the result of lifestyle.[11]

Today allopathic medicine continues its arrogant rejection and ridicule of acupuncture, chiropractic, osteopathy, and virtually all the alternative therapies that are almost always safer and more effective than a majority of drugs and surgical approaches.

Remember that science accepts as valid any treatment that produces results that are statistically significantly better than a placebo. Even if it is only 3 or 4% better than a placebo, and infinitely more risky, a treatment is considered useful.

Meanwhile, medicine and surgery go through fads, which are sometimes accepted for decades despite little proof of efficacy. Freezing the stomach for peptic ulcer is a case in point. Introduced by a guru of gastroenterology, it was, to my mind, probably no better than leeches. Even today such approaches continue. Despite the discovery that ulcers are partially caused by a germ and can be treated effectively with Pepto-Bismol or other safe, inexpensive medicines, most physicians still prescribe expensive and riskier therapy. Most people know now that George Washington was probably killed by purging and blood-letting–stupid and risky medical approaches in use less than two hundred years ago.

Twentieth-century medicine has its fads as well. Internal mammary artery ligation, the precursor of the modern coronary by-pass, was adopted with no double blind and no proof. Finally, a sham operation proved that the surgery was no more than a placebo. Imagine that! A simple incision in the chest cured 35% of patients with severe angina pectoris. The more radical operation of internal mammary artery ligation was only a placebo![12]

I could write an entire book on the useless fads that have fallen by the wayside. Just be aware that the "truth" of today may be exposed as a falsehood tomorrow. Even all the alternatives I mention may ultimately be replaced with better mousetraps. At least they are usually safe if you approach them wisely.

The vast majority of surgical procedures and drugs used today in Western medicine have been introduced in the past sixty years. Before 1939, the surgical procedures most in vogue today were not even imagined. A majority still have not withstood the test of science's gold standard, the "double-blind proof." Coronary bypass surgery, the greatest drain on medical resources, has become a fad in the past twenty-five years. Lumbar laminectomy, an operation generally prescribed for a presumed ruptured disc, was introduced just fifty-five years ago.

Antibiotics, tranquilizers, and other mood-altering drugs have evolved and have taken over medicine during the past fifty years. Anesthetics were unknown until 150 years ago, and virtually all of them in use today are recent additions.

At the beginning of this century, average life expect-

ancy was approximately fifty years; today it is roughly half
again higher. And 90% of that increase in longevity is the
result of improvement in the care of infants. Sadly, at the
same time, infant mortality in the United States is much
worse than that of other industrialized nations and even
that of many less-developed countries.[13] Some of the high
US infant mortality results from technological advances
that temporarily save premature infants who would have
been miscarried fifty years ago, but far too much is caused
by drug and lifestyle abuses of the parents. Although good
prenatal care lowers the infant mortality rate, smoking and
drugs are even more harmful than lack of such care.

Infections, the number-one cause of death in 1900,
were largely reduced by chlorination of water, proper
sewage disposal, pasteurization of milk, and adequate
supplies of protein. (The irony of chlorination is that it
does prevent infections, but causes other problems, as
discussed in Chapter 7.) Indeed, Dr. Thomas McKeown
has estimated that 92% of the improvement in longevity in
this century is the result of these public health factors.[14]

Only 8% of the improvement in length of life is the
result of our one-trillion-dollar disease treatment industry.
Indeed, Dr. Franz Ingelfinger, late editor of *The New
England Journal of Medicine,* stated:

> Let us assume that 80 per cent of patients have
> either self-limited disorders or conditions not
> improvable, even by modern medicine. The
> physician's actions, unless harmful, will therefore

not affect the basic course of such conditions. In
slightly over 10 per cent of cases, however, medical
intervention is dramatically successful, whether the
surgeon repairs bones or removes stones, the
internist uses antibiotics or palliative measures
(e.g., insulin, Vitamin B12) appropriately, or the
pediatrician eliminates a food that an enzyme-
deficient infant cannot absorb or metabolize. But,
alas, in the final 9 per cent, give or take a point or
two, the doctor may diagnose or treat inadequately,
or he may just have bad luck. Whatever the reason,
the patient ends up with iatrogenic problems. So
the balance of accounts ends up marginally on the
positive side of zero.[15]

Barely on the positive side of zero! Wow! Can you afford
modern medicine? When does it produce miracles? When
should you use modern medicine? The following symptoms are probably reasons to consult a physician.

Acute significant pain–especially in the head, chest,
or abdomen. The most common illnesses that *may*
require medical intervention to save your life or function are: meningitis, encephalitis, brain tumor, hemor-
rhage in or around the brain, heart attack (coronary
artery occlusion), pneumonia, appendicitis, and various
other obstructive or infectious illnesses in the abdomen.

Fever–especially above 100°F and not clearly related
to influenza. Some infections are quickly fatal, such as
meningococcal meningitis, abscesses, and several venereal

diseases. A fever higher than 104° may lead to brain damage. Other infections, such as TB, are much slower; in TB low-grade fever, especially with a chronic cough, may provide the warning signs.

Neurologic problems–Loss of consciousness, confusion, and partial or total paralysis are always indications for medical attention. Failure to act promptly may preclude recovery or limitation of disability.

Irregularity of heart beat–Some arrhythmias must be treated quickly. In general, only an M.D. or D.O. can decide what is indicated.

Bleeding–unusual or severe.

Swelling with or without redness or fever–medical judgment is needed for safety.

When in doubt, consult a physician–the life you save may be your own.

But there are many situations where medicine and surgery are *not* indicated and indeed can be dangerous to your health.

Anxiety–Unless you are truly panicked and overwhelmed, tranquilizers are not indicated. Relaxation, physical exercise, acupuncture, massage, photostimulation, and will power are all preferable.

Depression–Antidepressants may be indicated in fairly severe depression, but they always carry risks, as we will discuss in Chapter 9. At least 85% of patients can be safely, effectively, and more rapidly treated with alternative approaches. Incidentally, electroshock therapy is occasionally indicated, but perhaps only in a withdrawn, essentially vegetating depression.

When "nothing is wrong"—If a competent M.D. or D.O. cannot find a cause for your symptom, the likely problem is stress. If you are still worried, get an independent second opinion. Then, if you aren't satisfied, consider alternatives.

When you're told, "It's all in your head," the source of the difficulty is probably stress. There is no safe or effective medication or surgery for such problems. In that case, go alternative.

I could write a book attacking many aspects of modern medicine, such as unnecessary caesareans and many other surgical approaches, or the indiscriminate use of drugs. But there is nothing to be gained for you or me by such an approach. I am thus going to issue just a few warnings. Think carefully before you enter these therapies:

Elective surgery—If it's elective, it can wait, indefinitely—probably, permanently. Every anesthetic, every cut into your body is potentially fatal. Complications are common. Think more than three times and consider every conceivable alternative before you have elective surgery.

Insulin—Except in juvenile diabetes, insulin is rarely necessary. More importantly, far better control of adult-onset diabetes can be had with relaxation, good nutrition, adequate physical exercise, and the Ring of Fire/DHEA protocol.

Cortisone/Prednisone—Except in cases of adrenal fail-

ure, such as Addison's disease, chronic use of these powerful and very dangerous drugs is rarely needed. In acute
lupus erythematosus and temporal arteritis, these drugs
may be miraculously life-saving, but with chronic use,
they may prove equally life-threatening. I am appalled at
the frequent use of such powerful, risky drugs in rheumatoid arthritis, fibromyalgia, bursitis, and even
polyneuropathy. In virtually every such case, safe alternatives should be used before you risk your life and function.
DHEA is probably more effective and certainly far safer
than prednisone in any illness.

Chemotherapy–In only a limited number of cancers is
there clear-cut evidence of life-saving and enhancing
results from chemotherapy. Hodgkin's disease, lymphoma,
choriocarcinoma, and acute leukemia are the illnesses
where chemotherapy may be miraculous. Some breast
cancers also respond well to it. In virtually all other
cancers, patients suffer more and often die with many
more complications while undergoing chemotherapy.
Personally, I choose not to be poisoned. Instead, consider
some of the miracles of alternative procedures cited in this
book. (See Index for references to alternative cancer
treatments.)

Psychotherapy–Psychoanalysis is, from my perspec-
tive, perhaps the most glaring example of sick medicine.
Yes, patients do benefit, but statistically you'll do as well
contemplating your navel. Indeed, if you contemplate
your navel in a focused, meditative way, you'll do far
better. Except for psychotics, I question the value of the

entire field of psychiatry. Indeed, Freudian psychoanalysis has never been proven to be more effective than no therapy at all. Much of modern psychiatry is devoted to the use of tranquilizers and other mood-altering drugs, with very little counseling or education to get at the root causes. For most complaints of anxiety, guilt, anger, or depression, education and brief psychological counseling are much more effective than drugs. Jungian and humanistic psychologists do offer potentially useful therapy. There are almost unlimited alternative approaches worth pursuing for chronic problems involving the anxiety, guilt, anger, and depression resulting from unresolved fear, loss, or anger.

Besides, if you are motivated enough to read this book, you can probably care for yourself better than anyone else can do it for you.

STRESS–THE COMMON DENOMINATOR

Babies born to healthy mothers who have not suffered from German measles or taken drugs during pregnancy are almost always healthy. Medicine says the causes of illness can be classified in the following ways:

Hereditary–Hereditary (genetic) illnesses are both common and rare. That is, the gene gives a predisposition but usually not a destiny. Often, the incidence of such an illness in a person with a genetically related condition is only a few times greater than in those who lack such genes.

Consider epilepsy, for example. One percent of the population has epilepsy, but only 3% of those who have an

epileptic relative develop epilepsy. Even with the widely
touted recent discovery of a gene predisposing women to
breast cancer, only about 5% of women with breast cancer
have such a gene; the other 95% develop the disease from
other causes.

Congenital–A congenital disease is not genetic but
somehow acquired prenatally. Myelomeningocele, for
instance, is strongly associated–that is, in about 50% of its
victims–with maternal folic acid deficiency. This nutritional lack can be readily treated with vitamins before and
during pregnancy.

Vascular–Vascular illness is a term that is just a
pigeonhole; it does not imply cause. A problem with
arteries, veins, or capillaries is a major factor in causing
any vascular disease. But what caused the veins, arteries,
or capillaries to fail? Stress causes constriction and spasm
of blood vessels, as well as increased cholesterol and
ultimately atherosclerosis. Good nutrition, relaxation
therapy, and physical exercise can prevent most vascular
disease.

Degenerative–Degenerative illnesses are commonly
supposed to arise from wear and tear. Why doesn't everyone of the same age have more or less the same amount of
tissue degeneration? Although significant injury may
weaken an area, most degenerative illnesses, such as
osteoarthritis, do not have a satisfactory medical explanation.

Oncogenic–Oncogenic illness is a medical term for
cancers. By such a classification, cancer just "is." But

experts estimate that 85% of cancers are due to lifestyle. Probably, the other 15% are, too; we just haven't discovered the aberrant stress that causes it.

Traumatic–Traumatic illness occurs after an injury and certainly is a cause of some pretty difficult problems. But what caused the accident? At least 80% of persons involved in serious accidents were "care-less" because they were preoccupied with their mental chitta, the broken records of worry.

What medicine ignores, sadly, after sixty-plus years of marvelous research propelled by one of the unacknowledged heroes of research, Hans Selye, is the fact that all illness is the result of stress. *The key to health is stress management.* Without stress management, you will sooner or later experience disease. Without stress management, you will never achieve optimal health.

Stress by any other name is still stress, and it is *the* cause of illness. Stress management is the key to care of the self.

Now, to understand this fact, you need to understand stress. When the body experiences more pressure than it can handle naturally, it enters a state Selye called alarm. The alarm reaction may be caused by physical, chemical, electromagnetic, or emotional pressure.

Physical–The most obvious physical alarm is a cut or a fracture. Severe bruises are also obvious cause for alarm. Extreme temperatures (below freezing or above 90°F) are almost obvious. Not so obvious is physical inactivity–the couch potato syndrome. Going to bed for a week is as

stressful as breaking your leg. If you are unwilling to move
your body, you do not care about your holy temple.
*Nothing is more important or powerful in stress management
than physical exercise.* In general, this requires strenuous
exercise for three hours a week, at best, or if you move at
a slower pace, six hours a week. If you are not willing to
care for yourself to the tune of three to six hours a week,
then enjoy your illnesses. All the drugs and surgery and all
the alternative approaches in the world cannot equal the
value of adequate physical exercise in managing stress,
maintaining health, and in recovering from most illness.
Physical exercise is *the* antidote to stress. See my book,
The Self-Healing Workbook, for an overview of ways to use
physical exercise to manage stress.

Chemical–Chemical stress is, second only to physical
inactivity, our greatest cause of illness. Actually, in measurable terms, chemical stress causes well over 60% of all
illnesses. Tobacco, alcohol, and street drugs, as well as
consuming excess fat, salt, and sugar are prime chemical
stressors. In addition, too much coffee (more than two or
three cups a day) and virtually all sodas are stressors. Sugar
follows closely. Americans consume their weight in sugar
each year, but sugar has none of the vitamins or minerals
necessary for it to be metabolized.

Pollution is another major chemical stressor. From air
pollution to pesticides and herbicides, we are the most
poisoned people in history. Even chlorination of water,
which prevents many infections that occurred ninety

years ago, is not good for you. People who drink a normal amount of city water have an increased incidence of bladder cancer. The solution: filtered or spring water–an "alternative" that may not seem miraculous, but cutting the incidence of bladder cancer 50 to 66% by drinking filtered water is a near miracle.

Drugs, of course, are major chemical stressors. Most prescription drugs and all street drugs aggravate the total life stress. If a drug is not essential to your health or life, don't take it.

Electromagnetic energy–Electromagnetic or EM may be the most pervasive and least recognized form of pollution. Exposure to electromagnetic energy is harmful. It is now reasonably well known that continuous exposure to three milligauss of EM increases brain cancer and leukemia. EM is produced by all electrical devices (except the Liss cranial electrical stimulator and GigaTENS). Even "natural" electromagnetic energy is harmful at 35,000 feet–that is, in a jet plane. It is estimated that spending six hours in a plane at normal altitude is equal in chemical stress to smoking 200 cigarettes.[16]

Cars and their heaters, airplanes, typewriters, computers and especially printers, radios, electric clocks, waterbeds, televisions, fluorescent lights, and microwaves all produce tremendous amounts of abnormal, highly stressful electromagnetic energy. Stay as far as possible from such devices, especially as you sleep. Keep TV, radio, and electric clocks at least eight feet from your head.

Avoid electric blankets. Switch to a regular razor. Avoid hair dryers. Don't travel by air more than once or twice a month. I also recommend that you obtain a TriField Meter (available from Self-Health Systems) and test the various devices in your environment.

I feel that natural light and fresh air, always better for you than the caves we live in, is an antidote, or at least a partial antidote, to electromagnetic energy stress, and indeed it assists in all stress management.

The life/health you save may be yours or that of your loved ones.

Emotional–To most people, the very word *stress* means emotional distress–the reaction to fear. The most basic human fear is that of rejection or abandonment. Beyond this fear of loss of love, we also may fear death, being an invalid, or poverty, or we may be undergoing the existential crisis of meaning and values. Whatever the fear, our reactions are more or less limited to anger, guilt, anxiety, or depression. All the other negative emotional reactions are synonymous with these four.

In some aspects, the body/mind does not distinguish between causes of stress: physical, chemical, electromagnetic, or emotional. Whenever a stressor is enough to elicit an alarm reaction, the fight-or-flight response is an outpouring of adrenalin. Adrenalin causes the liver to release glycogen (stored glucose) to give more energy for the fight or flight; the hypothalamus/pituitary releases ACTH/ beta endorphins; the adrenals release cortisol and decrease production of DHEA (dehydroepiandrosterone), a change that leads to a decrease in production of estrogen and testosterone. Beyond this simple *primary* response to stress, a wide panorama of interactions ensues, bringing the entire electrical and neurological system into accommodation of the excess adrenalin–homeostasis, the natural balancing act.

Virtually all brain, mind, body, and emotional functions are dependent directly upon the chemicals produced by the nervous and endocrine systems. These chemicals may be produced in the brain itself, the peripheral nervous system, or the endocrine glands; and there is growing evidence that alteration of stimulus may lead to changes in one or more of the other. The feedback loops between the hypothalamic pituitary axis and their target endocrine organs are quite specific: ACTH stimulates the adrenals; excess or deficient ACTH leads to excesses or deficiency of cortisol production. Less reciprocal are the associated changes that occur in other organs and neurohormones: thyroid, estrogen, testosterone, and so on. Similarly, exogenous hormones, such as in birth control pills, have significant effects upon thyroid function as well as upon the pituitary.

It is probable that the ratio of testosterone to estrogen in men or estrogen to testosterone in women is critical to optimal sexual manifestation, although few studies have been reported. Mental, attitudinal, and emotional influences on neurochemistry have been less studied than their effects upon both hormonal and cellular aspects of immune function. But the immune system is equally influ-

enced by neurochemicals and neurohormones; indeed, it
is probable that primary modulation of immune function
is mediated by neurochemicals.

Many non-personal influences upon neurochemistry
have been reported, including light, temperature, color,
music, latitude/longitude, barometric pressure, exercise,
and time of day.

In addition to generating intrinsic emotional reactions, hypnosis has a powerful effect upon neurochemistry. And it appears that mental attitude may be more
important than specific sexual activity in determining the
neurochemical substrate. In a striking study done by the
Shealy Institute, four couples engaged in the privacy of
their homes in either masturbation, intercourse, or mutual
masturbation. Blood samples were drawn before the sexual
activity and fifteen minutes after. Beta endorphin, oxytocin, and prolactin went up markedly in six of the eight
subjects, with the *levels* of these chemicals highest when the
person most enjoyed the experience. In two individuals
who disliked masturbation, even though they agreed to
the testing, there were no changes. Even with intercourse,
less chemical response was seen in those who rated the
experience unsatisfying because of their attitude toward
the testing. The person who drew the bloods was not in the
house during the sexual activity.

The dominance of neurochemistry in mood, sleep,
behavior, pain, and immune function suggests that
neuromodulation of the neurochemical/neurohormonal
system is potentially of great clinical significance. Since

1976, we at the Shealy Institute have investigated the effects of very low amperage and safe electrical current upon a variety of neurochemicals, through the Liss cranial electrical stimulator and GigaTENS.

When the body is over-stressed, the return to normal may fail to occur and the body may overreact by developing hyperglycemia, thus leading eventually to burnout or exhaustion and all the diseases of adaptation. Selye demonstrated that repetitive or excess stress leads to adaptation, a state in which little reaction occurs with a given stress. But eventually, excess adaptation leads to maladaptation and diseases such as osteoarthritis, hypertension, asthma, allergies, and even cancer.[17] Ultimately all illness is the result of excess stress and the failure of natural homeostasis. When stress is extreme, the body breaks down instantly, as in fractures—which are a response to greater pressure than a bone can handle—to the instant peptic ulcer, which may occur with a burn, major injury, shot of cortisone, or emotional shock.

More commonly, though, stress is repetitive and cumulative. Indeed, Hans Selye said that every time we adapt to a stress, such as nicotine or caffeine, we lower the threshold for new stress—that is, our tolerance of new stress is lower. Thus, if one twin smokes, he or she will tolerate much less additional stress than the non-smoking twin.

Here are some estimates of the relative stress created by various stressors in virgin situations:

Pre Adaptation Daily Alarm Reactions

1 cigarette	1
1 cup of coffee	1
5 tsp. of sugar	1
1 donut	1
A fast-food milk shake	5
1 can caffeinated pop	3
1 can diet caffeinated pop	2
Regular use of white flour products	5
Drinking chlorinated fluoridated water	2
Living in a city of 50,000 population	1
Living in a city of 250,000 population	2
Living in a city of 500,000 population	3
Living in a city of a million population	4
Using pesticides/herbicides	4
Smoking 1 joint of marijuana	1
Being around a smoker all day	5
1-1/2 oz alcohol, 1 beer, 1 glass of wine	2
Being under ideal weight by greater than 10 lbs.	5
Being overweight 10–15 lbs.	5
Being overweight 16–25 lbs.	10
Being overweight 26–40 lbs.	20

More than 40 lbs. overweight	40
Taking no regular exercise	40
Taking only occasional physical exercise	15
Divorcing within last year	7
Sleeping for only 6 hours	4
Obtaining no regular relaxation	4
Being unhappily married	4+
Being chronically angry, depressed, guilty, or anxious	4+

If your daily stress exceeds ten total alarm points, you are at increasing risk of illness and premature death. And if your total daily stress amounts to twenty-five alarm points or more, you almost certainly have some evidence of adrenal burnout, with resultant low DHEA.

The single most critical chemical in the human is DHEA. Although the average is said to be 130–900 ng/dL in women and 180–1200 ng/dL in men, I find most adult women well below their optimal 550-980 and most adult men below 750–1250. In fact, even in a non-patient population of reasonably healthy adults, fewer than 10% display these healthy levels. Patients with chronic illnesses of almost any type have levels commonly below 220 and very often below 100. Only if the adrenals can be restored to normal function is health restoration possible.

Thus, if you want a simple barometer of your health reserves, get a fasting blood drawn for DHEA. Be sure it is sent only to Nichols Lab in Capistrano, CA (phone 800-553-5445). For more information on DHEA levels, see the chart on page 181, which shows the relation of DHEA to stress.

I believe that each of us has a genetic, constitutional health reserve. This reserve is used up by cumulative stress–physical, chemical, electromagnetic, or emotional. When a certain loss occurs, your weak spots begin to show up with symptoms or illness. Minor depletion may lead to generalized mild illness, such as susceptibility to a cold or influenza. Major depletion will lead to high blood pressure, heart disease, diabetes, or even cancer. Again, *every* disease is the result of total cumulative stress.

This pervasive aspect of stress is the reason so many different approaches may assist in relief of symptoms or apparent healing.

This is not to say that antibiotics are useless with stress-induced diseases. If you have meningitis, antibiotics may kill the stress-inducing bacteria, allowing the body to heal itself through homeostasis. Without antibiotics, healing of meningitis is rare; death is common. Such cures a hundred years ago would have been miracles.

With a ruptured appendix, surgery removes the infected appendix; antibiotics may help, and the body's homeostatic mechanism kicks in. (Before 1800, such a cure could have been a miracle.) With a majority of

DHEA and Stress

	Serious	Worrisome		Acceptable	
	Deficiency	Low	Fair	Good	Excellent
Male	<180	180-349	350-599	600-749	750-1250
Female	<130	130-299	300-449	450-549	550-980
	Exhaustion	Progressive Maladaptation		Adaptation	Homeostasis
	SERIOUS ILLNESS	DEGENERATION			

illnesses that can continue for months or years, however, only comprehensive stress reduction can allow healing. Thus in hypertension, although dozens of drugs might "control" or lower the blood pressure, none *cure* it. Similarly, coronary bypass surgery does not *cure* the disease of atherosclerosis; it temporarily unclogs one or more arteries.

The cure of hypertension or atherosclerosis requires alternative healing techniques. Thus acupuncture, through its effects on the electrical framework of the body, may be as effective as drugs. Nevertheless, long-term cure requires major stress reduction, such as that created by training the autonomic nervous system to avoid overreacting. Temperature biofeedback of the feet, weight balance, deep relaxation, and adequate physical exercise may cure hypertension totally. To allopathy, that is a miracle, for allopathic M.D.s often don't read the basic laws of science enough to accept them.

Similarly, atherosclerosis may be reversed–cured–by a low-fat diet, use of appropriate nutrients, physical exercise, and meditation. No drug or operation can accomplish this cure, an apparent miracle in light of medicine's failure to understand, accept, and, indeed, use this approach universally.

In certain illnesses, dealing with emotional stress may be adequate to reverse the disease. There is no one panacea for all illnesses, but there are many panaceas for each illness–in the form of stress reduction. Stress reduction, any way it is done, may allow the body to heal itself.

Thus faith and hope–the antidotes for anxiety–may be adequate for healing!

In general, the ten commandments for major stress management are:

- Avoid smoking
- Take no street drugs
- Consume a minimal amount of alcohol, or none
- Keep weight within 10% of ideal
- Minimize consumption of fat, salt, and sugar
- Exercise at least three hours and up to six hours per week
- Relax fifteeen minutes twice a day
- Sleep seven or eight hours per night
- Eat three meals a day of real food
- Resolve your anxiety, guilt, anger, and depression every day. Never go to bed with a grudge inside you or beside you.

NOTES

1. John Ott, *Light and Health* (Alpharetta, Georgia: Ariel Press, 1990).

2. Candace Pert, as quoted by Y. Baskin, "The Way We Act," *Science* 85 (November 1985): 96.

3. Stewart Wolf, M.D., "Disease as a Way of Life: Neural Integration in Systematic Pathology," *Prospectives in Biology and Medicine* 4(1961): 288–305.

4. Blair Justice, *Who Gets Sick* (Houston, TX: Peak Press, 1987).

5. *Ibid.*

6. E. Roskies, M. Iado-Miranda, and M.G. Strobel, "Life Changes as Predictors of Illness in Immigrants," in C. D. Spielberger and I. G. Sarason, eds., *Stress and Anxiety,* vol. 4 (Washington, DC: Hemisphere, 1977), pp. 3–21.

7. S.C. Kobasa, S.R. Maddi, and S. Courington, "Personality and Constitution as Mediators in the Stress-Illness Relationship," *Journal of Health and Social Behavior* 22 (1981): 368; S. R. Maddi and S. C. Kobasa, *The Hardy Executive: Health Under Stress* (Homewood, IL: Dow Jones–Irwin, 1984).

8. R.A. Good, "Foreword: Interactions of the Body's Major Networks," in R. Adler, ed., *Psychoneuroimmunology* (New York: Academic Press, 1981), p. xvi.

9. H. J. Eysenck, "The Respective Importance of Personality, Cigarette Smoking and Interaction Effects for the Genesis of Cancer and Coronary Heart Disease," *Personality, Individuality, Differences* 9 (1988): 453–464.

10. Eugene D. Robins, *Matters of Life and Death: Risks vs. Benefits of Medical Care* (New York: W.H. Freeman, 1984).

11. Thomas McKeown, *The Role of Medicine: Dream, Mirage, or Nemesis* (Nuffield, England: Nuffield Provincial Hospitals Trust, 1976).

12. E.G. Diamond, C.F. Kittle, and J.E. Crockett, "Evaluations of Internal Mammary Artery Ligation and Sham Procedure in Angina Pectoris," *Circulation* 18 (1958): 712–713; L.A. Cobb, G.I. Thomas, D.H. Dillard, K.A. Merendino, and R.A. Bruce, "An Evaluation of Internal-Mammary-Artery Ligation by a Double-Blind Technique," *New England Journal of Medicine* 260 (1959): 115–118.

13. Robins, *Matters of Life and Death:*.

14. McKeown, *The Role of Medicine: Dream, Mirage, or Nemesis.*

15. Franz Ingelfinger, "Health: A Matter of Statistics or

Chapter 9

Depression: From the Pits to the Peaks

And since you are a breath
in God's sphere,
and a leaf in God's forest,
you too should rest in reason
and move in passion.
–Kahlil Gibran

In no aspect of medicine have I seen more potential for miraculous improvement than depression. I believe that depression is the most prevalent illness in the world, as well as the most ignored. In recent years, more and more antidepressant drugs have been introduced; although they do help some patients, each drug is only about 40% effective if randomly assigned to depressed patients.

Perhaps it is worthwhile to begin with your analysis of yourself by means of the checklist below. Please be honest as you check the following list of the way you feel right now.

187

_____ Depressed mood.

_____ Losing interest or pleasure in things you used to enjoy.

_____ Experiencing significant weight change (loss or gain).

_____ Eating frequently between meals.

_____ Insomnia.

_____ Hypersomnia (sleeping too much).

_____ Sleepwalking.

_____ Feeling agitated.

_____ Experiencing sluggishness, slow to function.

_____ Fatigue, low energy, feeling tired all the time.

_____ Feelings of worthlessness or guilt.

_____ Difficulty concentrating, thinking, and remembering.

_____ Indecisiveness.

_____ Recurrent thoughts of death or suicide.

_____ Suicide attempts.

_____ Nervous exhaustion.

_____ Worrying excessively or being anxious.

_____ Crying frequently.

_____ Being extremely shy or sensitive.

_____ Being upset easily by criticism.

_____ Permitting little annoyances to get on your nerves and to make you angry.

_____ Getting angry easily.

_____ Becoming nervous around strangers.

_____ Feeling lonely.

_____ Having difficulty relaxing.

_____ Being troubled by frightening dreams or thoughts.

_____ Being disturbed by work or family problems.

_____ Wishing that you could get psychological or psychiatric help.

_____ Being tense or jittery.

_____ Being easily upset.

_____ Being in low spirits.

_____ Being in very low spirits.

_____ Believing that your life is out of your hands and controlled by external forces.

_____ Feeling that life is empty, filled with despair.

_____ Having no goals or aims at all.

_____ Having failed to make progress towards your life goals.

_____ Feeling that you are completely bound by factors outside yourself.

_____ Feeling sad, blue, or down in the dumps.

_____ Feeling slowed down or restless and unable to sit still.

_____ Suffering frequently from illness.

_____ Being confined to bed by illness.

Most people will suffer from one or more of these symptoms at some time. If you are now experiencing five or more of these symptoms, you are depressed, at least to some extent, and if you have at least fifteen other symptoms not related to mood, you are probably depressed. One of the huge problems with depression is that it is considered mental or emotional, and the medical insurance mafia discriminates against all mental illness, paying little toward therapy. Furthermore, antidepressant drugs,

when they work, require three to five weeks for effectiveness. And they all have some of the following significant
side effects: dry mouth, low or high blood pressure, weight
gain or occasionally loss, difficulties emptying bladder, or
sexual impotence.

Depression is just as real than any other disease
known. And it can be caused by a variety of factors, such
as:

- frequently interrupted sleep
- poor nutrition, including inadequate B vitamins,
  protein, or magnesium
- various hormonal disturbances, especially birth
  control pills
- pregnancy
- many drugs, including all tranquilizers, beta
  blockers, anti-hypertensives, anti-epileptics, di-
  uretics
- allergies of many types, including those to some
  foods as well as environmental pollutants
- anemia
- great stress, such as death of a loved one
- jet lag
- excess sugar or caffeine
- cigarettes/smoking
- alcohol
- inadequate physical exercise

- inadequate natural light
- any type of spiritual crisis
- DHEA deficiency

Of course, the *tendency* toward depression is sometimes inherited. Whatever the cause of depression, chronically depressed patients display more chemical abnormalities than do any other such people. These abnormalities include the neurochemical ones.

The nervous system manufactures and uses many chemicals. At least 92% of depressed patients have either excesses or deficiencies in from one to seven of the following:

Norepinephrine (NE)

Serotonin (ST)

Melatonin (MEL)

Beta endorphins (BE)

Cholinesterase (CHE) or the ratios:

NE/ST

ST/MEL

ST/BE

NE/BE[1]

If we add DHEA deficiency, commonly found in depression, all depressed patients have neurochemical abnormalities. When the depression is treated successfully, these abnormalities disappear. This DHEA deficiency may be responsible for the immune incompetency seen in depression.

A significant number of depressed patients respond positively to immunologic tests for rheumatoid arthritis, even though they have no major joint symptoms. And these positive rheumatoid factors clear up with relief of the depression. At least 78% of depressed patients are deficient in taurine, the most prevalent amino acid in the body. Taurine is essential for the stability of the electrical charge on muscle, nerve, or other cells. With an unstable membrane, all sorts of dysfunctions occur.[2]

Virtually all depressed patients are deficient in one or more of the essential amino acids, the amino acids we cannot manufacture but need to obtain from food. In fact, the neurochemicals listed earlier require some essential amino acid for their formation. Without these neurochemicals, widespread dysfunction is likely.

Among chronically depressed patients, magnesium deficiency is equally common, being found in virtually all of them. Unfortunately, most physicians don't even know how to test for magnesium deficiency. The serum magnesium test is useless except in cases of alcoholism and extreme nutritional deficiency; either a magnesium load test or an intracellular spectral analysis is needed for proper diagnosis.

Magnesium is involved in many enzymatic activities and also stabilizes membrane potentials. It works in harmony with taurine. At least 80% of women and 70% of men fail to eat even the recommended daily requirement of magnesium. In addition to accentuating depression, magnesium deficiency may contribute to heart attacks, high blood pressure, diabetes, cancer, and many other illnesses. Magnesium replacement, especially if done intravenously, may lead to near-miraculous clearing of depression.

The B vitamins are important for depressed persons, too. Deficiencies are common: 35% of non-smokers and 80% of smokers are deficient in Vitamin B6, a critical nutrient for brain and nerve function. Older people–those past sixty–are often deficient in Vitamin B12, too.

At least half of depressed patients are deficient in DHEA, dehydroepiandrosterone, the most prevalent adrenal hormone. Not one of more than one thousand depressed patients tested at the Shealy Institute has had *optimal* levels of DHEA (550 ng/dL or higher in women; 750 ng/dL or higher in men). Most chronically ill people–who are often depressed–are also deficient in this crucial hormone. In fact, 99% of chronically depressed patients have DHEA levels far below the optimal levels. DHEA is essential for health and longevity.

Depressed people may be deficient in other hormones including testosterone, estrogen, progesterone, and thyroid. Failure to check for these chemical imbalances obviously leads to failure to treat appropriately.

In addition to this vast number of chemical abnormalities, all depressed patients have one or more significant electrical abnormalities. On computerized EEG brain mapping, every depressed patient shows some asymmetry of the EEG, whereas, non-depressed people show almost identical quantities and qualities of electrical activity of the two sides of the brain. In 75% of depressed patients a strong focal increase in electrical activities appears in the right frontal lobe, with the other 25% of depressed people displaying the same asymmetry in some other area of the brain. The increased activity may be at any frequency: alpha, theta, delta or beta, and is unassociated with any abnormality on Magnetic Resonance Imaging or computerized x-ray scans.

When non-depressed patients are exposed to flashing lights (photostimulation), their brains increase electrical activity at the same frequency as that of the lights—that is, if they see ten flashes per second, the brain increases its ten-per-second electrical activity. In all chronically depressed patients there is no response, or there is a totally inappropriate response. These patients show increases to twenty per second or even decreases to three per second, with ten-per-second flashes.

Once the depression clears, the two sides of the brain show symmetry in electrical activity and eventually their brains follow photostimulation appropriately.

Over the past six years, I have worked with hundreds of chronically depressed patients who had failed to recover with one or more antidepressant drugs. I have been able to bring 85% of these patients out of depression within two weeks, without drugs and without undesirable side effects. In fact, most patients improve in other ways, eliminating many symptoms in addition to depression. These results represent one of the most consistent miracles of alternative healing. Because of my success in treating depression, I recommend the following treatments to be carried on simultaneously.

CRANIAL ELECTRICAL STIMULATION

Since 1976, I have used Saul Liss's cranial electrical stimulator (CES) to treat depression, as well as insomnia and some types of pain. The Liss CES leads to normalizing of beta endorphins and serotonin. In fact, 50% of depressed patients improve within two weeks using nothing else but an hour of CES every day, with no side effects. This treatment alone is much safer and more effective than any antidepressant drug.

One of the first patients I treated with CES came out of a sixteen-year depression within twenty-four hours of his first CES treatment—a true miracle at that time. Stimulation with the CES is not electroshock therapy. It uses only a thousandth of an amp of current, can be done at home by the patient without concern, and can be used even while eating, reading, or working. Even if no other alternative treatment were available, CES would still be the treatment of choice in all depressed patients. This device is the only part of the treatment that requires a physician's prescription in the United States; in most of the world, it is available over-the-counter.

PHOTOSTIMULATION

Since 1976, I have used photostimulation for assistance in

helping patients relax. We now know that photostimulation helps regulate beta endorphins, serotonin, testosterone, estrogen, oxytocin, and other hormones, as well as the EEG. For photostimulation we use the Shealy RelaxMate, a simple, inexpensive pair of goggles with two flashing lights, controllable for brightness and frequency (from 1 to 7.5 flashes per second) at the comfort level of the patient. We recommend using photostimulation fifteen minutes twice a day, plus an hour at night upon retiring.

EDUCATION

I have felt for many years that proper education is essential for optimal recovery. Through the years, our education program has been reduced to ten hours of lectures, and we have found recently that video-taped lectures work at least as well as live ones. Indeed, patients seem to remember more from the videotapes. Topics covered on the tapes include psychology and physiology of stress and mood, physical exercise, nutrition, psychological roots of hardiness vs. depression, a broad understanding of the metaphysical meanings of the body's energy centers, and spirituality. This videotape program is available for anyone from Self-Health Systems.

VIBRATORY MUSIC

Music has been used for centuries to calm the savage breast. In the Bible, David's soothing music calmed King Saul when he was in his fits of madness.[3] In recent years, music beds with built-in speakers have been used with great benefit both for helping patients relax and to release buried conflicts. We recommend an hour each day of vibratory music–hearing and feeling the music.

We have used Pachelbel's *Canon in D*, Beethoven's *Sixth Symphony*, Rachmaninoff's *Isle of the Dead*, Mozart's *Requiem*, Bearns and Dexter's *Golden Voyage #4*, Aeoliah's *Crystal Illumination*, Halpern's *Spectrum Suite*, and the *Best of Kitaro*. Recently, Ison's *Therasound* program has also seemed to offer excellent music for this therapy.

Commercially available music beds or chairs start at about $3,500, but you can build your own for about $1,000, including the cost of the stereo equipment. Music perceived in this way can provide a truly transcendent experience, and I find that the Therasound Harmonizing Tape moves chi in my body better than anything I've experienced except the GigaTENS, the latter not yet available to the public and probably a prescription item when it is released. Illustration 2 on page 198 shows a simple design for a music bed.

INSIGHT MEDITATION

Meditation of all types is helpful for everyone. The use of a special meditation chamber, however, provides an amplification unavailable in any other setting. The chamber is easily constructed, although it could be an entire room. See Illustration 3 on page 199 for a meditation chamber. The smallest version is fifty-four inches square and with

side walls forty-eight inches high. On each inside wall is a
three-foot-wide strip of smooth, shiny roofing copper,
backed by glass. One side is split in the center, with the
copper and glass split to allow entry. On top of the side
walls is a fifty-four inch copper tubing pyramid, the peak
of which reaches almost to the eight-foot ceiling of a room.
At the apex are placed two quartz and two amethyst crystal
balls, two and a half inches each in diameter. From the
apex hangs by a cotton rope a 250-gauss magnet, north
pole up, and the bottom of the magnet is lowered to within
six inches of the level of the top of your head as it is
positioned while you are seated on the floor. On the floor
is a lead sheet.

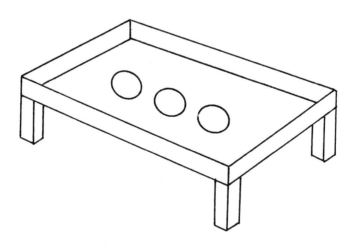

Illustration 2. The Music Bed

This chamber can be further amplified by applying a Tesla coil at any point on the copper. The Tesla coil puts out electrical energy at frequencies up to and including 78 billion cycles per second and charges the whole chamber with gigahertz. The coil is available from Electronics Products, Inc., 4642 Ravenwood, Chicago, IL 60640-4592. You need the model that can run continuously.

In such a chamber, a fluorescent tube will light up at any point at which it is placed, without its being attached to any fixture. Your entire body is then bathed in giga frequencies (up to 78 billion cycles per second, at one

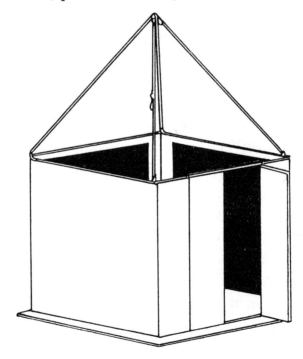

Illustration 3. The Meditation Chamber

billionth of a watt), which is a frequency similar to the
healthy vibrating frequency of human DNA. This chamber is safe for anyone except a person with a cardiac
pacemaker. It can be built for about $1,000 and provides
superb sacred space in which to meditate and allow
unfinished business to be released and resolved.

It is very useful for two persons who care for one
another and wish to work together to increase harmony.
We do not recommend that individuals at odds with one
another work together in the chamber.

Some individuals dislike the chamber immensely
because it gives them nightmares–really, "daymares"–
vivid and sometimes unpleasant imagery. Of course,
buried/suppressed anger, guilt, anxiety, and depression
are unpleasant when released. But such release is essential
to healing.

Some patients when they sit in the chamber experience remarkably creative imagery that appears spontaneously. Such creativity may be increased by using great
music, such as TheraSound, or by using a quartz musical
bowl, the resonance of which is greatly amplified in the
chamber. In fact, the vibration of the bowl is strongly felt
throughout one's body when it is played in the chamber.
The music bowl is highly recommended for those who
want to activate their highest potential. Quartz bowls are
available from Self-Health Systems.

How to Gain Insight

The meditation chamber provides an atmosphere in which

I believe lucidity is enhanced. Lucidity is the ultimate intuitive skill, in which you know the answer to a question. Sitting in the chamber, eyes open, looking at the slightly blurred image of yourself in the copper plate, your mind appears to be able to detach more easily from worry and receive intuitive answers or insights. Ask and you will receive, if you don't try too hard.

MAGNESIUM REPLACEMENT

Unless there is kidney failure, magnesium is safe in everyone and needed by most of us, even those not depressed. Ideally, depressed patients benefit rapidly from 10 shots of intravenous magnesium, each given over about 30 minutes. The IV consists of 50 cc. of IV fluid, with added 2 grams of magnesium chloride, 1 gram of calcium chloride, 250 mg. of dex-panthenol, 100 mg. B complex, 100 mg. B6, and 1000 units B12. For those who can't get the IV, we recommend 250 mg. (2 capsules) of magnesium taurate, best taken at bed time. It may take six months or more to replenish magnesium stores when it is given orally. If diarrhea occurs with oral magnesium, then it must be given intravenously. Those taking it orally should also take a 100 mg. B complex tablet daily. An oral spray of magnesium has recently become available. It can be ordered from Self-Health Systems.

AMINO ACIDS

Although taurine and most amino acids (except trypto-

phan, which is now banned, in my opinion unreasonably)
can be taken in tablet or capsule form, it is best to consider
meat broth as the medium because it provides all essential
amino acids. This broth is prepared by placing in a slow-
cooker or crock pot, 1 quart of water, 8 oz. of stew-sized
meat (such as chicken, turkey, fish, or beef), an onion, a
carrot, a stick of celery, 1 tbl. vinegar, and 1 tbl. soy sauce.
Cook this on low heat for 12 hours.

One could prepare a double recipe. For the first
month I recommend one quart of the meat broth daily;
during the second and third months, you should take one
pint, and then use one cup daily—forever. This is the best
way to prevent recurrent deficiency. Incidentally, there is
no vegetable source of taurine. My impression is that
depression is more common in vegetarians. Unless one
eats cheese or milk and eggs (lacto-ovo-vegetarian) I do
not recommend vegetarianism to anyone.

PHYSICAL EXERCISE

For anyone who is depressed, I strongly recommend
progressively increasing aerobic exercise. The goal is to
reach sixty aerobics points per week. You may require
three to six months to build up to this goal, but it is well
worth the effort. Such exercise is probably the single best
tool for preventing depression. There are many sources
for aerobic information, including my *Self-Healing Workbook*. The simplest formula is walking four miles in exactly
sixty minutes, which gives you eleven points. Four miles
in sixty minutes, five days a week, and two miles in thirty

minutes on the sixth day, thus gives you sixty aerobics points.

If you are pregnant, out of condition, or have heart disease, you should consult your physician about exercise. But if you can walk, it is safe to begin walking at whatever pace is comfortable for five minutes. Then each week add one or two minutes and build slowly to sixty minutes. When you can walk comfortably for sixty minutes, you can slowly pick up speed and aim for the levels mentioned above.

CRYSTALS

In 1988, we investigated the use of quartz crystal as an adjunct to healing depression. One hundred forty-one chronically depressed patients were randomly assigned double-blind (neither patient nor researcher knew which they got) either a glass crystal or a clear quartz crystal. The patients mentally programmed the crystal with their own healing phrase (see pp. 53–54 for discussion of the healing phrase), then wore the crystal in a pouch around the neck. Quartz (including amethyst, rose quartz, and herkimer) is piezo-electric, which means it can store and receive or emit electrical energy and transform physical energy into electricity. This principle is widely used in modern electronics. Theoretically, thought is electromagnetic.

At the end of our two-week intensive, 85% of the patients were markedly improved, whether they received glass or quartz. But with no further treatment, three to six months later only 28% of those who used glass remained

improved, whereas 80% of those who used quartz remained improved. This is highly statistically significant, at
the 0.001 level–meaning that there is less than one chance
in 1,000 that the quartz is ineffective. This performance
makes quartz considerably better than any drug! Is the use
of a quartz crystal a miracle? It certainly is beyond the
known laws of science.

Since 1989 we have routinely recommended that
patients use the quartz as a reinforcer. And in our latest
study, we still find 85% of those who use quartz crystals
improved when they finish the treatment program; moreover, 80% of those who watch the video education remain
improved.

THE SELF-HEALING WORKBOOK

This workbook was specifically created for my depression
research project. We give it to each patient at completion
of the two-week program, with an audiotape called *Rain-
bow Energy Balancing,* a guided imagery Biogenics exercise.
The workbook provides ninety-four days of specific physical, mental, emotional, and spiritual exercises. It is a
powerful tool for personal growth.

In a given year, thirty to sixty million Americans
suffer from depression, and I suspect that low-grade depression affects countless millions more. Anyone with
significant depression should have a counselor, therapist,
psychologist, minister, or physician as a guide while
working through depression. But on a program such as the

one outlined here, virtually everyone can move out of the pits and into joy within two weeks. Best of all, it is safe— faster and safer than any drug, more effective than any drug, and without risky side effects.

The program outlined in this chapter effects many miraculous cures. It provides long-term relief from depression to a higher percentage of patients than any other treatment. It is therefore clearly the treatment of choice for depression. Work with your therapist to include all the elements mentioned. I believe all chronic illnesses include depression; a spiritual or existential crisis is the root of most illnesses, and even when no apparent depression precedes a major illness, it often follows chronic failure to recover. Although drugs and surgery can provide critically important opportunities for cure in acute illness, they are rarely of great curative value in depression or chronic illness. The tremendous results achieved with the comprehensive, safe, alternative treatment program outlined here could revolutionize treatment of virtually all chronic illness.

NOTES

1. C. Norman Shealy, Roger K. Cady, R. G. Wilkie, Richard Cox, Saul Liss, and William Closson, "Depression: A Diagnostic, Neurochemical Profile and Therapy with Cranial Electrical Stimulation (CES)," *The Journal of Neurological and Orthopaedic*

2. C. Norman Shealy, Roger K. Cady, Diane Veehoff, Rita Houston, Mariann Burnetti, Richard Cox, and William Closson, "The Neurochemistry of Depression," *American Journal of Pain Management* 2 (January 1992): 13–16.

3. I Samuel 16:23.

Chapter 10

Alternative Care for Common Illnesses

Reason cannot see sin
but can see errors,
and leads to their correction.
—A Course in Miracles

> The difficult is not the impossible. . . .
> The conquest of difficulties makes up
> all that is valuable in earth's history.
> —Aurobindo

Example is not the main thing
in influencing others. It is the only thing.
—Albert Schweitzer

> If all the pharmacopoeia in the world
> were thrown into the ocean,
> it would be to the betterment of humanity
> and the worsening for the fishes.
> —Sir William Osler

You *can* create your own miracles, especially if you assist them with faith, hope, and self-esteem. Every thought is a prayer, and your carefully focused thoughts and prayers can lead to the miracle of true healing. However, you should also take advantage of the practical miracles of alternative medicine, wise nutrition, and healthy living set forth in this chapter. If you truly expect a miracle, you will prepare for it by gathering all the resources of mind, body, and spirit. Then you can joyfully accept your miracle.

You may, however, have to fight fiercely to find assistance in choosing some of the alternative treatments I've outlined here. In general, holistic physicians are more likely to assist you. Holistic nurses sometimes function as facilitators. Family physicians, especially those trained recently, are more open than most medical/surgical specialists. Osteopathic physicians and chiropractors tend to be more open to alternatives than M.D.s. Humanistic psychologists are much more open than most conventional psychologists; to get in contact with one, write the Association for Humanistic Psychology, 45 Franklin Street, #315, San Francisco, CA 94102. Unity, Science of Mind, and Religious Science ministers are generally wonderful resources for assistance.

When your physician "can't find anything wrong," tells you "it's nerves" or "in your head," or recommends a tranquilizer, you should search carefully for alternative options. With chronic illness or serious illness, in addition to consulting your physician, I strongly recommend a second opinion from a holistic physician and careful consideration of these alternative options. The life you save or the miracle you create may be your own.

For all the therapies outlined in this chapter, if your physician will not assist, consult the American Holistic Medical Association, 4101 Lake Boone Trail, Suite 201, Raleigh, NC 27607.

Below is an alphabetic list of health problems with my recommendation for their treatment. Many of these approaches may seem too medical or technical for you. These are my own personal alternative protocols. Any holistically oriented physician will understand any terms you do not know. Also, most of the terms are explained or discussed elsewhere in this book; please consult the index for assistance.

The guidelines given here simply provide a place to begin your discussion with a physician. If your physician is unwilling to be helpful and consider safe alternatives, then switch health practitioners.

ADDICTION–DRUG, TOBACCO, ALCOHOL

Therapy

The basic need is a major stress reduction therapy.

Step I

    A. Deep relaxation at least 20 minutes, twice a day. Audiotapes from Self-Health Systems help.

    B. Progressive vigorous physical exercise, building to at least 1 hour, 6 days a week.

    C. Good nutrition.

    D. The following will need a cooperating physician.

       1. Cranial electrical stimulation 1 hour daily for 4 weeks.

       2. Acupuncture–ear and/or body.

       3. Lithium orotate 45 mg. per day.

       4. Tryptophan 1 gm. (or 5-OH Tryptophan 100 mg.) 4 times per day plus 4-6 gm. at bedtime plus 100 mg. B complex per day. US readers should check with your holistic practitioner about the tryptophan, which is currently banned by the FDA.

       5. Gamma hydroxybutyrate 4 gm. at bedtime.

       6. Melatonin 6 mg. at bedtime.

       7. Trans-Mins Complete Mineral Formula 2 per day.

       8. Symmetrel 100 mg. 3 times per day.

       9. Brain synchronization with a Shealy Relax-Mate for at least 15 minutes 4 times per day.

Step II

If the above program is inadequate, we recommend the two-week intensive Biogenics program at the Shealy Institute plus six months follow-up hypnosis and counseling, including Past Life Therapy.

AGITATION/SEVERE ANXIETY/PANIC

Evaluation

The usual medical and comprehensive psychological evaluation. Check magnesium level and DHEA. Avoid tranquilizers!

Therapy

Step I

    A. Cranial electrical stimulation.

    B. Daily dose of 45 mg. lithium orotate.

    C. Try gamma hydroxybutyrate 750 mg. 4 times per day with niacinamide 1 gm. 3 times per day.

    D. Consider Desyrel 25 mg. 4 times per day.

    E. Magnesium IV as per protocol.

    F. Build up to 60 aerobics points per week as rapidly as is safe.

    G. Massage.

    H. Acupuncture, especially the treatment for "non-violent madness."

    I. Transcutaneous electrical nerve stimulation (Electreat–use on hands and/or the top thoracic vertebra to sacrum).

    J. Hypnosis, especially with Past Life Therapy and counseling.

    K. DHEA supplementation, if deficient.

L. Start on the audiotapes *Balancing Body Feelings* and *Balancing Emotions* (both from Self-Health Systems), 4 times per day, plus use of the brain synchronizer at beginning of therapy.

M. Brain synchronization for 15 to 30 minutes, 4 to 8 times per day.

N. Two-week Biogenics program at the Shealy Institute.

Step II

Consider Buspar, but only temporarily while aiming for other therapy to put an end to the problem.

AIDS

In our book, *AIDS: Passageway to Transformation,* Caroline Myss and I report one "white crow," a young man who actually recovered from AIDS. The miracle of his recovery appears to have been accomplished by the nurturing acceptance of his family and the "Sea Salt Meditation" recommended by Caroline.

In addition to the general recommendations for enhancing immune function, in this illness I recommend dehydroepiandrosterone (DHEA), at least 250 mg. 4 times a day to raise DHEA levels to at least 750 ng/dL.

ALLERGIES

Evaluation

Consider including Epstein-Barr Virus testing in the workup if fatigue is prominent.

Therapy

1. Avoid, for 1 month, all wheat, corn, eggs, dairy, citrus.

2. Vitamin C (calcium ascorbate): build to 15 grams per day plus zinc picolinate 60 mg. per day, selenium 100 micrograms per day, Trans-Mins Complete Mineral Formula 2 per day, and samolinic oil capsules 9 per day.

3. Castor oil packs to the abdomen daily for 1 month.

4. Try Echinacea, 5 drops 4 times per day and Ligusticum, 5 drops 4 times per day.

5. Organic germanium, 3 tablets per day.

6. Biogenics tapes *Balancing Body Feelings* and *Balancing Emotions,* 4 times per day.

7. Build to 60 aerobics points a week.

8. Sunlight 2 hours a day.

9. Check your DHEA and follow the DHEA/Ring of Fire protocol.

ANOREXIA AND BULIMIA

Evaluation

The major evaluation is psychological, but you should also check amino acid profile, intracellular magnesium, and DHEA.

Therapy

1. IV magnesium for 10 days.
2. Use the Liss CES 1 hour each morning.
3. Brain synchronization.
4. Intensive 2-week Biogenics training at the Shealy Institute.
5. Hypnosis and Past Life Therapy.
6. Basic allergy diet.
7. Build to 75 aerobics points per week.
8. Weekly hypnosis and/or counseling for 6 months.
9. Meat broth at least 2 cups per day for 1 month and 1 cup per day indefinitely.
10. Replace DHEA if deficient.

ASTHMA

Evaluation

Standard medical evaluation; intracellular magnesium; DHEA.

Therapy

1. Magnesium IV for 5 to 10 days and usual allergy program.

2. Two-week intensive Biogenics program and brain synchronization.

3. Acupuncture.

4. DHEA supplementation if deficient (virtually all will be).

AUTOIMMUNE DISORDERS AND IMPAIRED IMMUNE SYSTEM–PSORIASIS, RHEUMATOID ARTHRITIS, CANCER, EPSTEIN-BARR VIRUS (EBV), CANDIDA

Evaluation

Essential to do DHEA testing.

Therapy

1. IV Vitamin C–50 grams with 100 mg. B6, 1 gm. calcium chloride, 2000 mg. magnesium chloride in 500 cc's 2.5% D/W. Try 5 days, but may be needed for 2 plus weeks.

2. Castor oil packs to abdomen times 1 month plus twice a week for 6 months.

3. Sunlight 2 hours per day.

4. Avoid dairy, wheat, eggs, corn, citrus for 1 month.

5. Try macrobiotic or No Added Fat Diet.

6. Food supplements as for allergies.

7. Biogenics 2-week intensive with hypnosis, Past Life Therapy, counseling, brain synchronization.

8. DHEA supplements and Ring of Fire protocol.

9. *Nutrition to Improve Immunity.* Eat two meals a day of raw fruits, vegetables, nuts, and seeds, choosing those you like and enjoy. Eat one meal a day of brown rice, steamed vegetables, and broiled, poached, or steamed fish. Season with herbs.

Basic Daily Supplementation:

Beta carotene (not Vitamin A!)	Up to 200,000 units
Vitamin C (build up slowly)	Up to 2-5 grams
Vitamin B6 or B Complex	100 mg.
Magnesium (Mg Taurate is best)	125 mg. 2 times a day
Zinc	30 mg.
Pycnogenol	30 mg. 2 per day

You may add:

Selenium	100 mcg.
Vanadium	50 mcg.
Chromium	1 mg.
Copper	1 mg.
Echinacea	5 drops, 4 times a day
Ligusticum	5 drops, 4 times a day
Astragalus	1 capsule, 3-4 times a day
Shiitake mushroom	1 capsule, 4 times a day

Generally, vitamins should be taken with food, and minerals can be taken on an empty stomach. Do not take magnesium along with calcium or with a meat meal. Be sure your diet contains plenty of fresh vegetables.

You should also be sure to get essential fatty acids. The best supplement is a samolinic oil capsule, a combination of approximately 0.5 gram of salmon oil and 0.5 gram of a quality vegetable oil (borage, flax, or primrose). I recommend 6 oil capsules, a day.

For examples of miracle healing with diet read *Cancer–50 Cases* by Max Gerson. I believe the diet I've mentioned to be easier to use than the one Gerson recommends, and just as good.

The Seuterman homeopathic approach may be useful, especially in autoimmune problems. It requires physician planning.

10. *Castor Oil Packs.* It has been shown that castor oil on the surface of the body does enhance immune function even in normal people.[1] Since I consider castor oil so important, here are the instructions.

Materials Needed

    a. flannel cloth

    b. plastic sheet–medium thickness

    c. electric heating pad

    d. bath towel

    e. two safety pins

Instructions for Use

Prepare a soft flannel cloth (preferably wool flannel, but cotton flannel is all right if wool is unavailable). The cloth should be two to four thicknesses and measure about 10 inches (25 centimeters) in width and 12 to 14 inches (30 to 35 centimeters) in length after it is folded. This is the size needed for abdominal application. Other areas may need a different size pack. Pour some castor oil onto the cloth. This can be done without soiling the bed if a plastic sheet is underneath the cloth. Make sure the cloth is wet but not drippy with the castor oil. Then apply the cloth to the area that needs treatment.

Next, apply a plastic covering over the soaked flannel cloth. (HandiWrap is excellent.) On top of that, place a heating pad, set at medium to begin with, then turned up to high if the body tolerates it. It may help if you wrap a towel, folded lengthwise, around the entire area, and fasten it with safety pins. The pack should remain in place for an hour or an hour and a half.

The skin should be cleansed afterward by using water prepared as follows: To a quart of water, add two teaspoons of baking soda. Use this to cleanse the abdomen. Keep the flannel pack in a plastic container for future use; it need not be discarded after one application.

Frequency

You may use a castor oil pack 4 times a day and you may even sleep with it.

Castor Oil Suits

You can make a castor oil "suit" for the entire body. For the average person who is using castor oil for detoxification, re-energizing, or immune system enhancement, I recommend using 3 or 4 ounces of castor oil. Begin by taking a shower and drying off. Spread 3 or 4 ounces of castor oil gently and liberally over the entire body, from the ankles right up to the neck. Spread particularly thickly around the abdomen. Then put on then a pair of long johns or a fleece-lined jogging suit. The best are gray jogging suits that sometimes have a white lining, which make them extra thick. Sleep in this. Take it off the next morning. Your skin will be soft, but not greasy, and most of the time you don't even have to take another bath and can go on with your daily activities. The cloth suit may be used two to three evenings, but by then it needs to be washed, because the oil will begin to come through the surface.

For those people who also have abdominal problems and want the total body suit plus the pack, I recommend the following: Place another 2 ounces of castor oil on the abdomen itself, following the directions for the castor-oil pack, then go ahead and apply the castor oil body suit. This will give the abdomen an extra dose of castor oil.

You should use castor oil packs or suits at least once a week; twice a week is better. For people who are having acute problems or chronic moderately severe problems, I recommend their use every night for 1 to 4 weeks, and then twice a week.

CASTOR OIL BATHS

I have found castor oil baths to be energizing and probably beneficial for enhancing the immune system function, although there is yet no scientific substantiation of this. There is good substantiation that castor oil packs of the abdomen do enhance immune function.

To take a castor oil bath, fill the tub with moderately warm water, hot enough for a good soak. You are going to stay there from 20 to 30 minutes. The water should cover the entire body up to the top of the neck when you lie in the tub. When the tub is about half full, take one-half cup of castor oil, place it under the running water, and then slosh it around very vigorously, to mix the oil as much as possible with the water. When the tub is appropriately filled, get in the tub and rub your body gently all over, to be sure that the oil is deposited on every part of the body.

After 20 or 30 minutes, when you are ready to get out of the tub, drain the water completely from the tub. Then wash your body twice, scrubbing thoroughly with at least four ounces of any good shampoo, but *do not stand up!* The tub will be dangerously slippery. You may sit in the tub with the shower running over you, or rinse off with the faucet running. Once you have thoroughly washed and rinsed yourself twice, crawl out and over the edge of the tub onto a bath mat; *do not try to stand in the tub.* Immediately afterward, wash out the tub *thoroughly* with shampoo, scrubbing every square inch of the tub to be sure all oil is removed.

Dry off, and then rest covered with a light sheet, at least until your body temperature returns to normal.

11. *Saunas and Heat Therapy.* A sauna has been said to be highly useful in helping the body sweat out some environmental contaminants, and it is well known that this type of heat enhances certain aspects of immune function. Sit in the sauna for 45 to 90 minutes, with the temperature at 105° to 115° F.

To undertake any heat therapy, one should always be in reasonably good shape and should drink plenty of extra water. It is worthwhile taking a thorough bath afterwards. Probably the body is best washed with a good quality shampoo, since it cuts skin oils better than regular soaps do.

12. Use the Shealy RelaxMate, the photostimulator mentioned earlier.

Cancer

Scientists are finally beginning to recognize that an ability to find cancer at an early stage may not be important. Dr.

H. Gilbert Welsh of White River Junction, Vermont, states, "We are heading down a very slippery slope." Although 39% of women between the ages of forty and fifty who die of non-malignant disease are found at autopsy to have microscopic evidence of cancer in the breast, in fewer than 7% of women does cancer become clinically diagnosable. Therefore, with our current detection methods, only 1% of women in that age range will have been diagnosed clinically as having cancer. Dr. William Black of Dartmouth University states that there is very good reason to believe that many very early cancers never become clinically significant.

Parasites and Cancer

A unique new concept in the field of alternative treatment for cancer is the one reported by Hulda Regehr Clark, Ph.D., N.D., in her book, *The Cure for All Cancers,* ProMotion Publishing, 1993.

Dr. Clark, who has a Ph.D. in physiology from the University of Minnesota and a naturopathic degree, believes that cancer is caused by a parasite, the human intestinal fluke, *Fasciolopsis buskii.* She believes that there are other parasites that also cause disease, including the sheep pancreatic fluke and many others. Ordinarily the liver would trap and kill the parasites, but she believes that propyl alcohol—which is found in a variety of products ranging from cold cereals to shampoo to toothpaste—disables the liver from performing this vital function.

Dr. Clark also states that seizures are caused by

Ascaris; schizophrenia and depression by parasites in the brain; asthma by *Ascaris* in the lungs; diabetes by the pancreatic fluke of cattle, *Eurytrema;* migraines by the thread worm *Strongyloides;* acnae rosacea by *Leishmania;* and that much human heart disease is caused by the dog heartworm, *Dirofilaria.* She states that AIDS is caused when a parasite–usually the intestinal fluke–infests the thymus gland.

She believes that the flukes are present in raw meat, in saliva, in semen, in blood, in mother's milk, in urine, and, of course, in our pets.

Dr. Clark takes an unconventional approach to medical testing. The most important test for cancer, in her opinion, is the test for orthophosphotyrosine in urine. She believes that protein 24 antigen is the test for HIV. In conventional medicine, one would look in the stool for parasites, but Dr. Clark tests the white blood cells. This is a totally non-standard way to look for parasites, especially an intestinal fluke. She does perform a muscle biopsy to diagnose toxoplasmosis.

It is much too early to evaluate the validity of Dr. Clark's findings and recommendations. On the other hand, the treatment program itself is extremely safe, and I refer you to her book for the specific initial parasite-killing program, as well as a maintenance program. If I had cancer, I would certainly try her approach along with enhancing the immune system.

She believes that three herbs can rid you of more than a hundred types of parasites without so much as a headache or nausea. These three are: black walnut hulls (the hulls must be prepared from the green state), wormwood from the *Artemisia absinthium* herb, and common cloves. The cloves kill the eggs, while the wormwood and black walnut kill adult and developed middle life cycle stages of the parasites. Although she claims that cures are sometimes effected in as little as five days, patients must take these herbs for life in a maintenance program. She lists a hundred cases with brief reports of cures using her regimen.

CARPAL TUNNEL SYNDROME

Evaluation

Clinical examination; intracellular magnesium; DHEA.

Therapy

1. No smoking or caffeine.
2. Trans-Mins Complete Mineral Formula 3 per day for 6 weeks; then 2 per day for 6 weeks; then 1 per day.
3. B6 1000 mg. per day for 6 weeks; then 600 mg. per day for 6 weeks, then 300 mg. per day for 2 months; then 100 mg. per day.
4. If this fails in 6 weeks, consider steroid injection and, only if that fails, surgery.
5. Consider CES, black on forehead, red on palm, 60 minutes in the morning.
6. DHEA, if deficient.

CHOLESTEROL, ELEVATED

Evaluation

Standard blood tests, including HDL cholesterol.

If you eat as I have recommended, relax 30 minutes per day, exercise adequately, and still have a cholesterol level above 200, I recommend the following regimen.

Therapy

1. Stress reduction: a minimum of 15 or 20 minutes of deep relaxation twice a day.

2. Get adequate physical exercise, which means roughly the equivalent of walking 4 miles in 60 minutes 5 days a week, and 2 miles in 30 minutes on the sixth day every week. Other exercises can be done that would take somewhat less time, but walking gives you the equivalent quantity of cardiovascular exercise needed. As always, you should start slowly and build up over 3 to 6 months.

3. Avoid animal fats, except butter. All margarines are artificially hydrogenated, making them "bad" fats. About 1 tablespoon per day of butter is not bad. There is excellent evidence that both olive oil and canola oil (especially uncooked) in the amount of 1 or 2 tablespoons a day can assist in lowering cholesterol.

When all of the above fail, the most beneficial treatment is to consume the following:

- Timed-release niacin, 500 mg. twice a day.
- Cholestratin, 200 mg., 3 tablets twice a day.
- Acidophilus capsules, 500 mg. twice a day.
- Charcoal tablets, 260 mg., 8 to 10 tablets twice a day if the above fail.

Some people can get by with taking just a little bit more of any one of these; or the combination will work well. The only way you can find out in the long run is to check your cholesterol and test it after being on a regimen for a month.

People who take timed-release niacin should have their liver enzymes checked occasionally, since timed-release niacin may change liver function tests. Although generally that is not a significant problem, it should be kept in mind.

Only if, despite all these measures, your cholesterol is above 350, should you consider taking one of the cholesterol-lowering drugs. All drugs for lowering cholesterol carry significant risks.

CORONARY HEART DISEASE: ANGINA PECTORIS AND HEART ATTACKS

Evaluation

EKG and an Eliot cardiac stress test. I do not recommend a treadmill. It may precipitate a heart attack.

Prevention

The best approach to this most common illness (and most common cause of death) is prevention. Prevention is simple and remarkably effective.

- Avoid smoking and tobacco use.
- Keep your weight within 10% of ideal.
- Exercise adequately: 60 aerobics points per week. A discussion of aerobics points is included in Chapter 9 under "Physical Exercise."
- Relax 15 to 20 minutes twice a day.
- Take the recommended food supplements.

Such safe and simple life habits will cut the risk of heart disease at least 80%.

Dr. Dean Ornish has demonstrated reversal of hardening of the arteries with a simple, safe program of physical exercise, meditation, and a low-fat diet. In addition, the cholesterol-lowering program mentioned earlier is worth consideration.

Once heart disease develops, with angina pectoris as one major warning symptom, these habits, and perhaps cutting your fat intake to 10% of your total calories, will still help at least as many people as will coronary bypass surgery! Personally, I'd also consider 20 chelation treatments in this situation. Properly done, chelation is quite safe, although conventional medicine foolishly rejects it.

Chelation has probably saved thousands of lives and improved the quality of life for many more. It requires an intravenous injection over a 3 to 4 hour period once or twice a week.

With an acute heart attack, the treatment of choice is intravenous magnesium. If you are at risk of heart disease, find yourself, in advance, a physician who is willing to be sure the first consideration is intravenous magnesium. Beyond that, an acute situation requires proper conventional treatment. But once you recover from the acute problem, move immediately to the preventive program–except the 60 aerobics points. Begin exercise by starting to walk as long as you are comfortable–not over 15 minutes. Build gradually to an hour 6 days a week. Then work on speed. And as with all serious illness, measure your DHEA and begin rejuvenation of the "Ring of Fire" as soon as possible.

Therapy

1. Magnesium load.
2. 2-week intensive Biogenics training at the Shealy Institute.
3. Build to 60 aerobics points/week–walking only until up to level. This process may take 6 to 12 months.
4. Olive oil, 1 tablespoon per day.
5. Samolinic oil capsules, 6 per day.
6. Life Support pills, 3 per day.

7. Magnesium taurate, 125 mg., 2 at bedtime.

8. Transcutaneous electrical nerve stimulation.

9. Acupuncture.

10. Lifelong Biogenics 4 times per day and brain synchronization.

11. If cholesterol is elevated, see natural ways to reduce cholesterol (see: Cholesterol, Elevated).

12. Check DHEA and follow the DHEA/Ring of Fire protocol.

DEPRESSION

Depression is the most common symptom known and is the foundation upon which most illnesses develop. Underdiagnosed and poorly treated by conventional medicine, depression is cured by alternative medicine 85% of the time.

Evaluation

The usual medical and comprehensive psychological evaluation. Check magnesium level and DHEA.

Therapy

1. CES (cranial electrical stimulation). This totally safe device should be used routinely in every case of depression, applied 40 to 60 minutes each morning between 6 A.M. and 9 A.M. It requires a prescription. If your doctor won't prescribe it, find another, or come to the Shealy Institute for a 2-week program.

2. Photostimulation with the Shealy RelaxMate, 15 minutes twice a day and an hour at bedtime.

3. Vibratory music in the music bed (see Chapter 9) 1 to 2 hours per day, playing such music as Mozart's *Requiem*, Beethoven's *Sixth Symphony*, *The Best of Kitaro*, or David Ison's *Therasound*.

4. Meditation in the Insight Meditation Chamber (see Chapter 9) for an hour every day.

5. A 10-hour video program, "Vision, Creativity, and Intuition," provides the education we have found effective. It covers all essential aspects of nutrition, exercise, and psychological concepts of healing. You can order it from Self-Health Systems.

6. Food supplements. See the first six supplements listed under "Autoimmune Disorders."

7. Drink meat broth: a quart a day for a month, a pint a day for the next two months, then a cup a day forever. Almost all depressed patients are deficient in from one to eight of the essential amino acids. You don't have the building blocks to restore your body without them.

8. Exercise is essential; you should build up to 60 aerobics points a week. Both mental and physical exercise are crucial to the depressed person.

9. If DHEA is deficient (it will be!), supplement for 3 months at 100 mg. twice a day, while stimulating the Ring of Fire with the Liss CES.

For a detailed view of effective alternative treatment for depression, see *The Self-Healing Workbook* (Shealy, Element Books, 1993).

If you are on antidepressants, don't stop suddenly. Find yourself a therapist to guide you on this critical path.

DIABETES

Evaluation

At any age, diabetics should start with measurement of DHEA and restoration of the "Ring of Fire."

Therapy

Step I

1. Good nutrition—a wide variety of real food with lots of fiber.
2. Physical exercise—60 aerobics points per week.
3. Deep relaxation 20 minutes twice a day. This lowers insulin requirement up to 50%.
4. DHEA restoration.

Step II

If Step I is inadequate, follow this regimen:

1. No Added Fat Diet: consider avoiding dairy, wheat, corn, eggs, and citrus the first month.
2. Build to 75 aerobics points per week.

3. Begin Biogenics tapes *Balancing Body Feelings* and *Balancing Emotions* 4 times a day, plus brain synchronization.

4. Hypnosis with Past Life Therapy.

5. Two-week intensive Biogenics training at the Shealy Institute.

6. Consider zinc picolinate 60 mg. per day and chromium GTF 1 mg. per day.

7. Consider magnesium intravenously for 2 weeks.

Step III

If all the above treatments fail, try the Barnes Diet. It is discussed in detail in *The Self-Healing Workbook..*

DYSPAREUNIA

Evaluation

Dyspareunia is vaginal pain during sexual intercourse. A thorough pelvic exam is essential to rule out organic disease or other conditions. The only extra tests needed are intracellular magnesium and DHEA.

Therapy

1. Two-week intensive Biogenics training at the Shealy Institute.

2. Past Life Therapy and counseling.

3. When patient is aroused but before intercourse, gently penetrate the vagina with a finger or a candle in a condom.

4. Spouse and patient counseling.

EPILEPSY

Evaluation

The usual medical, neurological, and EEG evaluation. Also, test intracellular magnesium, amino acid profile, and DHEA.

Therapy

1. Trans-Mins Complete Mineral Formula 4 per day.

2. Taurine 1000 mg. 3 times per day.

3. Brain synchronizer (Shealy RelaxMate) at least 2 hours a day.

4. Biogenics tapes *Balancing Body Feelings* and *Balancing Emotions* 4 times a day with brain synchronizer.

5. CES transcranially 40 minutes a day for 2 to 4 weeks.

6. EEG biofeedback training.

7. Past Life Therapy.

8. Melatonin 12 mg. at bedtime.

9. Acupuncture.

10. If EEG is normal after 6 months free of seizures and on comprehensive treatment, consider slow weaning from anti-convulsants.

GALLSTONES

Evaluation

An ultrasound of the abdomen.

Therapy

The best treatment is a liver flush. Many variations are available. I prefer the one described in Jethro Kloss's *Back to Eden.*[2]

The liver flush is preceded by several days of an apple-juice fast. Then on the evening of the flush, take a mixture of 4 ounces olive oil and lemon juice. Although I am not aware of any complications of this approach, theoretically a large stone might move and block the bile duct. You should always be prepared to see a surgeon if severe pain develops.

HIGH BLOOD PRESSURE

Healthy individuals of any age normally have a blood pressure of approximately 120/80. Hypertension is diagnosed when blood pressure is 150/90. Thus, when the systolic pressure exceeds 140 and the diastolic exceeds 88, you need to take measures to bring it down. Both strokes and heart attacks are more common in those with hypertension.

Hypertension is a reaction to stress, so deep relaxation is an essential need. Remember that deep relaxation for 10 minutes twice a day decreases adrenalin production 50% for the entire 24 hours. Perhaps the easiest method for deep relaxation is to lie on the floor with your calves on a chair, thighs at right angles to the floor and calves. Stretch your low back to flatten it on the floor, then reach up and stretch your neck to flatten it and place your arms at right angles, as in the "stick 'em up" position. Breathe slowly and deeply, concentrating on nothing except breathing.

At the same time, you can say to yourself with each breath in, "My feet" and with each breath out, "are warm," while imaging the sun pleasantly warming your feet and allowing yourself to feel the pulsation of your heartbeat in your feet. Buy yourself a small thermometer, tape it to your big toe, and check the skin temperature at the beginning and end of this exercise. When you consistently warm your toes to 96° F, you will probably have good control over your blood pressure. This simple biofeedback tool is effective in 80% of patients with hypertension—one of the miracle alternative treatments. Even more critically, I recommend measurement of DHEA and stoking the "Ring of Fire" to restore adrenal homeostasis.

Two other great adjuncts are to be certain you get at least 1000 mg. of calcium and 500 mg. of magnesium each day. Most hypertensives are low in both these essentials.

Physical exercise is also terrific for stress reduction and stabilization of blood pressure. All hypertensive drugs have a huge variety of risky side effects, ranging from impotence to confusion. Although control of hypertension is essential for health and longevity, the simple, safe alternatives are likely to work if you do them.

For some hypertensive individuals, homeopathy, acupuncture, and herbs offer alternatives worth pursuing.

Evaluation

Along with the usual medical evaluation, check intracellular magnesium and DHEA.

Therapy

1. Intravenous magnesium for 10 days.
2. Add Trans-Mins Complete Mineral Formula 3 a day for 4 to 6 weeks.
3. Try samolinic oil capsules, 1 gram each, 9 a day.
4. Lithium orotate 45 mg. plus B-complex 100 mg. per day for 3 to 4 weeks.
5. Build to 75 aerobics points per week.
6. Hypnotherapy.
7. Restrict sodium intake.
8. May begin Biogenics tapes *Balancing Body Feelings* and *Balancing Emotions* 4 times a day in the morning.
9. Consider De-Tense herbal remedy.
10. Brain synchronization 15 minutes 4 times a day.

If the above approach fails, consider two-week intensive Biogenics training at the Shealy Institute. Especially learn to warm feet to 96° F. You must continue for 6 months.

LUMBAGO

Perhaps the most useful term for low-back pain, *lumbago*, is not commonly used today. Nevertheless, it may cover this most prevalent human complaint better than the term *back strain*. Unfortunately, conventional medicine has ignored since about 1939 the traditional term and concepts.

Low-back pain, with or without sciatica (radiation of pain down the leg), is the leading cause of worker's compensation claims and, until the advent of coronary bypass surgery, led to the most commonly performed surgery, laminectomy. As early as 1972, I reported that at least 90% of all lumbar spine operations for so-called ruptured disc should not be performed. Indeed, I suspect that 99% may not be needed.

Basically, low-back pain is most often due to muscle spasm, often with minor mechanical dysfunction or sprain of one or more facet joints, the small joints on either side of each vertebra posteriorly. The second most common cause is a sprain of the sacroiliac joint, which actually is a large facet joint. Muscle spasm creates pain, which causes more muscle spasm, thus perpetuating a cycle of pain. A ruptured disc may be as rare a cause of lumbago as metastatic cancer or osteoporosis. Although degenerative arthritis is common, especially at the lower two lumbar vertebrae, it is not the common cause of significant low-back pain.

Unless there is concomitant weakness of the foot or skin numbness of the big toe or side of the foot, there is no need to be worried about urgent intervention. And even with these two neurologic signs and symptoms, a ruptured disc is less common than nerve pressure from muscle spasm.

Nevertheless, when significant acute lumbago begins, it is wise to have regular x-rays of the lumbosacral spine–to have a baseline and to rule out the most serious concerns of metastatic cancer or a compression fracture from osteoporosis. And when there is nerve impairment (numbness or weakness), MRI (magnetic resonance imaging) is indicated. Only if there is a definite significant rupture of a disc, with at least 50% weakness of dorsiflexion of the foot, is surgery indicated. Even then, I would opt first to try intravenous colchicine, 1 mg. a day for 4 or 5 days. At least 75% of ruptured discs can be cured with this simple and, if properly done, safe procedure. The injection must be done slowly into a vein in the antecubital (front of elbow) fossa. For this I prefer a 24-gauge Jelco plastic needle. Using this approach I've seen even a 75% foot drop miraculously disappear within 48 hours. If you have a ruptured disc and your physician won't use colchicine, find another physician! After initial clearing of the neurologic signs and pain, you should remain on colchicine, 0.6 mg. per day, orally, and you should add two grams of Vitamin C and 100 mg. of B complex per day.

When there is no ruptured disc (a "bulging" or "protruding" disc is not ruptured), then the treatment of choice in lumbago is TENS, transcutaneous electrical nerve stimulation. Properly applied, TENS provides gratifying relief in 80% of patients with acute lumbago.

When TENS is inadequate, the next treatment of choice is acupuncture. Sir William Osler, the father of American Medicine, considered it in 1912 to be the treatment of preference. It is a wonderful treatment and may provide instantaneous, miraculous relief of pain; miraculous since conventional medicine's laws fail to account for its benefits.

When TENS and acupuncture fail, one or two treatments by an experienced D.O. or chiropractor who performs manipulation, may provide instant relief. If there is no striking improvement within three treatments, manipulation is no longer worth consideration.

The next line of defense is injection of Marcaine, a local anesthetic, under x-ray image intensification into the facet joints and/or sacroiliac joint(s) in the area of pain. This procedure is more likely than manipulation to be of benefit when the back pain has been present for more than 6 months. When two such simple temporary nerve blocks relieve the pain, then a permanent procedure using 1/2 cc. of 4.5% phenol in glycerine has an 80% chance of providing permanent relief.

Beyond these procedures, the treatment most likely to work is a combination of intravenous magnesium, corrective exercise, and retraining the nervous system or Biogenics.

In severe osteoporosis, calcitonin injections may be of help. At least three weeks of treatment are necessary to determine possible benefit.

In osteoarthritic pain, spinal or otherwise, it is worth trying glucosamine 500 mg. three times a day for 1 month and continuing if it helps. If glucosamine fails, then try shark cartilage 750 mg., 12 capsules per day for 3 weeks and continue at 6 a day if it helps greatly.

In acute lumbago, ice packs may help. In chronic situations, ice and/or heat may be useful.

Non-steroidal anti-inflammatories, modern or traditional (aspirin!) may be helpful but, as with all drugs, they have a significant incidence of side effects—undesirable and potentially serious complications. Acetominophen is, in my judgment, useless. Recently we have found wild yam root capsules (15 to 20 per day) excellent for osteoarthritic pain. (They are available from Self-Health Systems.)

MENOPAUSAL SYMPTOMS

Menopausal symptoms are probably not the cause of your mood swings, hot flashes, and night sweats if DHEA is above 550 ng/dL. There are alternatives to hormone replacement.

Evaluation

General medical and pelvic examinations.

Therapy

1. Daylight for 2 hours a day without glasses.

2. Get adequate physical exercise: build to 60 aerobics points per week.

3. Follow usual good health habits, especially the addition of magnesium to the diet.

4. Deep relaxation 20 minutes twice a day.

5. Photostimulation 20 minutes twice a day and an hour at bedtime.

6. Acupuncture with an experienced acupuncturist (Tchong Mo activation).

7. Herbs–Herbal-F, 1 in the morning and 2 in the evening.

8. If DHEA is less than 550, use ProGest cream (available from Self-Health Systems), 1/4 teaspoonful twice a day, applied to breasts and surrounding skin. If it is below 300, use the Liss cranial electrical stimulator to the Ring of Fire along with the ProGest.

MIGRAINE

Evaluation

Migraine is a vascular headache triggered by many factors. A headache specialist trained by Dr. Cady of the Shealy Institute is ideal for doing the evaluation. Interestingly, a majority of migraine headaches occur during barometric pressure changes or the approach of weather fronts. Check DHEA and intracellular magnesium. Check the neck for possible facet contribution. Consider food sensitivities.

Acute Management

Try the following treatments, one at a time.

1. Use Imitrex. If it is not effective in 30 minutes, try the following remedies.
2. Acupuncture.
3. Use the Liss cranial electrical stimulator.
4. Apply ProGest Cream to the skin, up to one tsp. at the onset and over the next hour.
5. Use an ice hat.

If the above fail to affect the migraine, next time try dihydroergotamine, 0.5 mg. injected intramuscularly.

Chronic Management

All the following treatments may be started together.

1. If DHEA is below 550 ng/dL, use ProGest cream, 1/4 teaspoon twice a day, as above. If below 300, use the Liss cranial electrical stimulator on the Ring of Fire, along with ProGest.
2. Use temperature biofeedback to train yourself.

3. If intracellular magnesium is low, take magnesium taurate 125 mg., 2 capsules at bedtime.

4. Use acupuncture weekly for at least six weeks.

5. Use the Liss cranial electrical stimulation daily, as well as at onset of headache.

6. Avoid foods you may be allergic to. For one month avoid milk, citrus, wheat, corn, and eggs.

7. Use deep relaxation, 20 minutes twice a day and an hour at bedtime.

8. Photostimulation 20 minutes twice a day and at onset of headache. Use the low intensity light.

9. Check the neck for possible facet contribution. Consider facet nerve blocks during a headache.

10. Try one aspirin a day.

11. Try 9 grams of evening primrose oil or samolinic oil daily.

12. Try feverfew, 400 mg., 1 capsule 3 to 4 times per day, or feverfew tincture, 6 to 8 drops 2 to 3 times per day.

13. Build to 60 aerobics points per week.

14. Be sure to use good health habits:

    No smoking

    Adequate sleep

    Good nutrition

    Resolve your anger, guilt, anxiety, or depression.

Additional Therapy

1. *Nutritional Approaches.* Many foods can trigger migraine, including Chinese foods (monosodium glutamate), red wine, cheese, chocolate, and in some individuals wheat, corn, citrus, eggs, or milk. At least 60% of patients can minimize migraine by avoiding all these foods and adding them back one at a time.

    Try the following:

    *   Tryptophan, currently banned by FDA but available in turkey, bananas, and peanuts. One may still get it in Canada. Three grams at bedtime may stabilize blood serotonin levels.

    *   Lithium, a small amount of lithium aspartate, 5 mg. three times a day; or lithium carbonate (a prescription compound) 150 mg. a day.

    *   Evening primrose oil and salmon oil–6 to 9 gm. per day.

    *   Magnesium: magnesium taurate three times a day is worth considering, if twice-daily doses fail.

2. *Temperature Biofeedback.* One of the safest and most effective tools for controlling migraine is the use of temperature biofeedback; 84% of patients improve and control headaches by learning to warm the fingertips to 96°F. This is

accomplished by practicing the control 3 times a day, for 15 minutes each time, measuring the finger temperature while relaxing and:

- repeating over and over "My hand is warm."
- imaging the sun pleasantly warming the hand.
- feeling the pulse in the fingers.

From three to six months of practice is necessary.

3. *Brain Synchronization.* Using photostimulation, such as the Shealy RelaxMate, for 15 minutes 3 times a day, and at the beginning of a headache, can reduce the frequency and severity of migraine by 80%. But it does require consistent practice for from 3 to 6 months.

4. *CES.* Cranial electrical stimulation can relieve migraine if used at the onset of a headache; red in front, black in back; or use the bi-temporal; or mastoid/nape of neck (red) to the muscle area between thumb and index finger. Daily use may serve as a preventative.

5. *Acupuncture.* Many migraines can be stopped by acupuncture, and continuing therapy may control future attacks.

6. *Acupressure.* Apply deep physical pressure at the nape of the neck, over the facet joints between the second and third cervical vertebrae for from 30 to 60 seconds; apply similar pressure to the muscle between the thumb and index finger; and

to the roof of the mouth, just behind the upper front teeth. Repeat up to 3 times for each attack, as early as possible.

7. *Facet Nerve Blocks.* Local anesthetics applied on the facet joints at C2-3 as early as possible after the onset of a headache may completely relieve the pain.

   If on 2 occasions complete headache relief is obtained, denervation of the joint may be considered, using 0.5 cc's of 4.5% Phenol in glycerine. Obviously, this procedure requires a physician well-trained in the technique.

8. *Drugs.* In general, the best drug for acute management is sumatriptan (Imitrex). In the 25% of patients who fail to respond to it, consider:

   • Lidocaine (100 mg. IV with 25 mg. Benadryl)

   • Mexitil–400 mg. by mouth at onset of headache, in an adult

   • Lithium carbonate–as mentioned earlier

I disapprove of the use of beta blockers, anticonvulsants, narcotics, and tranquilizers.

9. *Other Nerve Blocks.* Occasionally trigger spots at the base of the skull or in the neck can relieve a headache.

10. In intractable headaches, migraine or tension-related, a two-week Biogenics session at the Shealy Institute is strongly recommended.

MYOFASCIAL PAIN SYNDROME
(FIBROMYALGIA)

It appears that a majority of individuals who suffer from incapacitating myofascial pain develop it following a traumatic event of some kind. The event may be an automobile accident or a lifting accident at work, and it seems to be associated with a significant or potentially significant fear reaction. The fear may upset serotonin and norepinephrine balance. It may well be that a failure to express the anger or fear by screaming or fighting back helps to aggravate the situation long-term. Sufferers may then feel guilty over the need they feel for revenge and feel angry or violent toward themselves as well as toward others when they can't accept these feelings. Is it possible that the adrenalin surge created by such thoughts leads to a suppression of beta endorphins and interferes with sleep, perpetuating a vicious cycle? This situation would almost always be aggravated by magnesium deficiency, and magnesium deficiency is aggravated by major traumatic events and by an excess of adrenalin production, or norepinephrine production. DHEA deficiency is typical in fibromyalgia.

Evaluation

Check especially for osteopathic problems and depression; intracellular magnesium; DHEA.

Therapy

All these treatments are done concurrently.

1. Trans-Mins Complete Mineral Formula 3 per day.

2. Samolinic oil capsules, 1 gram, 9 per day.

3. CES 40 to 60 minutes a day for 12 weeks, 30 minutes transcranially and 30 minutes to the Ring of Fire.

4. Daily peanut oil massage.

5. Comprehensive limbering exercises.

6. Build to 60 aerobics points per week.

7. Lithium aspartate 45 mg. a day; 100 mg. B-Complex a day.

8. Gamma hydroxybutyrate 4 gm. at bedtime.

9. Melatonin 6 mg. at bedtime.

10. Hypnosis.

11. Biogenics tapes *Balancing Body Feelings* and *Balancing Emotions* 4 times a day.

12. Sunlight 2 hours a day.

13. Consider Elavil, Desyrel, or Ludiomil.

14. DHEA, 100 to 200 mg. twice a day.

15. Consider a two-week intensive Biogenics training.

OSTEOPOROSIS

Evaluation

X-ray confirmation is essential. DHEA evaluation and

intracellular magnesium.

Therapy

1. Boron 3 mg. per day.
2. TENS, CES, and/or acupuncture as appropriate.
3. No Added Fat Diet.
4. Consider trial of IV vitamin C 50 gm. per day (for pain only).
5. Trans-Mins Complete Mineral Formula 3 per day.
6. Consider Calcimar, 100 micrograms daily for 3 months and then 2 to 6 per week.
7. Build to 75 aerobics points per week.
8. Biogenics tapes 4 times a day.
9. Two-week intensive Biogenics program at Shealy Institute if pain is severe.
10. ProGest cream, 1/4 tsp. twice a day.

PAIN CONTROL

The Shealy Institute has been the leading American chronic pain clinic for almost 25 years. The following is a summary of our philosophy developed in helping at least 85% of more than 10,000 chronic pain patients.

Drugs

In general, drugs are not only of little or no help but they prevent natural body balancing (homeostasis).

Narcotics

Demerol; morphine; Percodan; codeine; Empirin #2, 3, or 4; and Dilaudid are all narcotics. As such, they are:

> addicting,
>
> habituating,
>
> of little value after 2 to 4 weeks, and
>
> require increasing dosages.

They do sedate or narcotize more than they produce analgesia or pain relief. Under almost all circumstances they should not be used for more than a month.

Tranquilizers

Valium and almost all tranquilizers convert anxiety to depression. They block both Stage 4 and REM sleep. They make patients irritable, depressed, or fuzzy-thinking. They block the normal endorphin restoration stage. They should not be used more than a month.

Narcotic Agonists/Antagonists

Darvon, Talwin, Stadol, and Nubain, in my opinion, are useless and addicting. They block endorphin receptors and lead to depression. These drugs should never be used except in acute situations. More critically, they should never be used at the same time narcotics are given.

Aspirin and Acetominophen

Aspirin is the best analgesic for acute and chronic use. Except in rheumatoid arthritis, no more than 12 tablets a day should be used. For those with a sensitive stomach, timed-release aspirin, Ascriptin, or Magan may be useful. If it helps and does not cause stomach pain or bleeding, aspirin may be taken indefinitely.

Acetaminophen, in my experience, is a poor substitute for aspirin; use it only for those who are truly allergic or have stomach intolerance of aspirin.

Ibuprofen and some of the newer anti-inflammatory drugs are occasionally worthwhile. They usually have a higher incidence of complications than aspirin. Our favorites are Orudis, Naprosyn, Lodine, and Ansaid. Aleve is the best over-the-counter anti-inflammatory drug.

Antidepressants

All chronic pain patients have some level of depression. Elavil is one of the better of the antidepressants. Small dosages help restore Stage 4 sleep and are especially useful for that purpose. Moderate dosages (150 mg.) help depression and may help pain. About 25% of patients cannot take Elavil because of complications (dizziness, dry mouth, confusion, drowsiness, agitation, and low blood pressure, for example).

Most other antidepressants have even more complications and rarely work as well as Elavil. There is little evidence that Limbitrol, Surmontil, and Sinequan are as useful as Elavil. Tofranil may be.

Desyrel is excellent for sleep assistance. Remember, it may cause priapism in males—an inability to lose erection.

Zoloft, Effexcor, Paxel, and Wellbutrin are worth considering, if necessary.

I consider Prozac more dangerous than any other antidepressant except monoamine oxidase inhibitors. Monoamine oxidase inhibitors are indicated only in severe depression, usually under a psychiatrist's supervision. They must not be taken with tricyclics, such as Elavil.

Cranial electrical stimulation (CES) usually works as well as antidepressants. Indeed, the program outlined in the depression chapter should be your *first option.*

Phenothiazines

In extreme agitation Thorazine may be useful for a short period of time. It sedates better than most other tranquilizers. Many complications are possible, and it is used for a few weeks or less in desperate situations.

Vistaril and Librium

As temporary sedatives, especially to assist in drug withdrawal symptoms, these drugs may have a beneficial effect. Usually, they are not required for more than a month.

Sleeping Pills

These are not for chronic use. All sleeping pills—Placidyl,

Dalmane, Halcion, chloral hydrate, Seconal, Nembutal, Doriden—are addicting or habituating. They prevent restorative or Stage 4 (endorphin-replenishing) sleep. They should be used not more than 1 week under desperate circumstances. They may require slow withdrawal. If cranial electrical stimulation fails to work, consider the Shealy RelaxMate. And if necessary, use GHB (Gamma Hydroxybutyrate) 500 mg. up to 4 grams at bedtime, with 6 to 12 mg. melatonin.

Drug Withdrawal

Narcotics, narcotic antagonists, and tranquilizers can be withdrawn over a period of from 7 to 12 days, usually without symptoms. CES is most valuable in preventing withdrawal symptoms. Use the depression treatment protocol.

Colchicine

Intravenous colchicine may help low-back pain, acute ruptured discs, and pain of arachnoiditis (inflammatory spinal scar). It is given daily for five days concomitant with oral colchicine (0.6 mg. per day or it can be 1 mg., 3 mg. on two days). If a good result is not obtained within five days, it should be discontinued. Although it can affect blood production or cause nausea, complications are rare. Continue taking orally for 6 months or longer if it proves helpful.

Food Supplements and Nutrition

Many patients with chronic pain eat a terrible diet. Furthermore, under chronic stress some essential nutrients are needed in greater quantity. Consider the first six supplements mentioned in the "Autoimmune" section.

Caffeine

Caffeine is a stimulant like a weak shot of adrenalin. In chronic pain, caffeine aggravates the pain. All forms of caffeine (colas, tea, coffee, Empirin, Anacin, and Excedrin, for example) should be minimized.

Nicotine

Nicotine is, in my experience, the worst offender, possibly worse than narcotics, for patients with chronic pain. It causes spasm of blood vessels; blocks an essential body chemical, Prostaglandin E_1 (PGE_1); and lowers magnesium reserves. When PGE_1 is blocked, inflammatory scarring is more pronounced, and the immune system is weakened. About 90% of patients who fail to get well after back surgery are smokers!

The good news is that pain may recede rapidly when smoking ceases. See the section above on "Addiction" for details.

Sugar

Table sugar, corn syrup, and other sugars deprive the body of essential vitamins and minerals. They should be minimized.

White Flour

White flour, even "enriched," is deficient in vitamins, minerals, and fiber. It places extra metabolic stress on the body.

Fats

High levels of fat (40% of calories in the average American diet) are associated with increased heart disease and cancer of breast and colon. Trans-linoleic acid–produced in artificially-hydrogenated fats, such as Crisco, all margarines, solid vegetable shortening, smooth peanut butter, and artificial creamers–interferes with PGE_1 production and should be avoided.

Tryptophan and B Complex

Tryptophan, with vitamins B3, B6, and lithium, is converted to 5-hydroxytryptamine, or serotonin. Disturbances of serotonin metabolism may lead to irritability, insomnia, depression, and pain.

In dosages of from 3 to 10 grams per day, tryptophan works at least as well as sleeping pills and antidepressants, without significant side effects. A few patients experience nausea because of the large number of capsules; a few need to take the last dose 4 or 8 hours before bedtime. If you have trouble sleeping with tryptophan at bedtime, the last dose may be taken about noon or by 2 P.M. Unfortunately, in the United States the FDA banned this safe, effective nutrient! One can get it in Canada.

Along with the tryptophan, 100 to 200 mg. of B complex should be given. It has been reported that a huge majority of chronic pain patients are deficient in one or more B vitamins.[3] Blood tests may confirm this, but it is less expensive to give trial supplements for 4 to 6 weeks.

Tryptophan is usually tapered off after 4 to 8 weeks.

Vitamin C

Chronic pain patients who are smokers may be deficient, or borderline, in vitamin C levels. A trial of from 1 to 3 grams per day may be worthwhile.

Greenwood has reported that vitamin C is quite helpful in healing patients with symptoms of ruptured disc.

Phenylalanine

Both 1- and d-phenylalanine have been reported to be useful in patients with chronic pain. D-phenylalanine blocks enkephalinase.

From 3 to 4 grams per day may be tried for up to a week. If there is no response by then, it should be discontinued. It should be given only after withdrawal from narcotics, tranquilizers, and sleeping pills.

Evening Primrose Oil/Salmon Oil

When inflammation of muscles or nerves is present, samolinic oil, 1 gram, 3 times per day, may be helpful in stimulating PGE_1 production.

Minerals

Chronically ill patients may be deficient in many minerals, including calcium, magnesium, zinc, chromium, manganese, and lithium. Laboratory tests for these are not as clear-cut as desired. Hair analysis coupled with blood tests may be helpful in this situation. But the Trans-Mins formula, 3 per day, should be adequate.

Magnesium

Seventy-five percent of Americans are clearly deficient in magnesium, and 9% are borderline. This difficulty comes from deficiency in the food supply and in absorption. The magnesium load test is the most efficient and accurate in measuring for deficiency. Intracellular magnesium testing is the test of choice. Have your physician contact Intracellular Diagnostics at 1-800-874-4804 for information.

Sleep

Inadequate sleep (fewer than 7 or 8 hours, or lack of Stage 4 or REM sleep) may cause pain, usually of a generalized nature but often concentrated in back, neck, and head (fibromyalgia).

Sleep restoration is assisted by:

1. Withdrawal from caffeine, sleeping pills, nicotine, and tranquilizers.

2. Adequate physical exercise–45 to 60 aerobics points a week. See details below.

3. Cranial Electrical Stimulation (CES). Safe and highly effective CES often restores a normal sleep pattern within a week or two. It should generally be given for 30 to 60 minutes daily before 1 P.M.

4. Gamma Hydroxybutyrate, 4-5 gm. at bedtime. An excellent "natural" hypnotic, available on prescription through Thayer Pharmaceutical, 1101 E. Colonial Drive, Orlando, Florida 32803, 800-848-4809 or from Apothe'Cure, Inc., 13720 Midway Rd., Suite 109, Dallas, TX 75244, 800-969-6601.

5. Melatonin 6 mg. at bedtime helps some but not all patients.

6. Biogenics (mental self-regulation) is highly effective in reducing stress, assisting relaxation, and maintaining homeostasis. Mental self-regulation exercise is a major assistant in restoring normal sleep patterns.

7. Transcutaneous Electrical Nerve Stimulation (TENS) can be used to assist relaxation by

passing current intensely between the palms for about 20 minutes or passing the positive current at the top of the thoracic spine, negative at the sacrum.

8. Brain Synchronization with the Shealy Relax-Mate often induces adequate relaxation at 3.1 hertz to assist in going to sleep.

Physical Modalities

1. *Heat/Ice; Whirlpool.* Both heat and ice may reduce pain. An empirical trial is worthwhile. Whirlpools provide an opportunity for total body relaxation.

2. *Acupuncture.* Fifty percent of patients with chronic pain are improved by acupuncture. From 10 to 25 treatments may be necessary. In acute pain, 80% of patients are improved. The initial trial should be 3 treatments.

3. *TENS.* Fifty percent of chronic pain patients and 80% of acute pain patients achieve 50 to 100% pain reduction with properly used TENS. TENS (and acupuncture) does not work well when patients are taking narcotics, narcotic antagonists, or tranquilizers. Extensive exploration of output variations may be necessary to optimize results. When combined with the Shealy System of audiotapes, 80% of chronic pain patients improve from 50 to 100 percent.

4. *Massage.* Total body and facial massage assist relaxation and limbering. Muscle spasm may be reduced by massage.

5. *Nerve Blocks.* Nerve blocks may be diagnostic or therapeutic. Nerve blocks may be done with a local anesthetic (Novocain, Xylocaine, Marcaine, Calphosan, or Sarapin). Almost any nerve can be blocked, but nerve blocks are impractical in generalized pain. From 10 to 30 nerve blocks may be necessary to achieve lasting relief. Mixtures of Calphosan, Marcaine, and Sarapin are useful for desensitization. Trigger point and facet nerve blocks are most helpful. In chronic pain, epidural blocks rarely provide long-term relief and are much more risky. We do not administer them.

6. *Physical Exercise.* No single treatment is as good as proper physical exercise. This includes:

   Limbering–full range of motion (stretching) all muscles, joints and tendons.

   Strengthening–of weak muscles.

   Conditioning–aerobics exercise increases oxygen consumption and heart rate and stimulates beta-endorphin production. No other treatment is as effective for depression and for pain control. From 45 to 60 aerobics points are required for good pain control. It takes 3 to 6 months to build up to 45 or 60 points. Example: Walking 4 miles in 59 minutes = 11 points.

PEPTIC ULCER, COLITIS, AND OTHER GASTROINTESTINAL PROBLEMS

Evaluation

Standard medical evaluation and x-rays are essential.

Therapy

Begin with the first four techniques; if they fail to give relief, continue to the fifth treatment.

1. General stress reduction, such as the comprehensive stress reduction program outlined earlier.

2. Castor oil packs to abdomen 3 times per day for 1 week, then 2 times per week for 6 months.

3. Biogenics tapes *Balancing Body Feelings* and *Balancing Emotions* 4 times a day.

4. Hypnosis and Past Life Therapy.

5. Consider 2-week Biogenics training at the Shealy Institute if the previous treatments don't work..

PHANTOM LIMB PAIN

Evaluation

Standard medical evaluation.

Therapy

Try each of these treatments, one at a time.

1. Consider intense acupuncture and TENS to stump.

2. If no immediate effect, try acupuncture and TENS to contralateral similar areas.

3. Gamma hydroxybutyrate up to 4 gm. per day, lithium orotate 15 mg., B-Complex 100 mg. daily, all at least for 1 month.

4. D-/L-Phenylalanine 4 gm. per day for at least 3 weeks.

5. Consider series of desensitizing nerve blocks into trigger spots on stump.

6. Cranial electrical stimulation head to stump.

7. If all the above fail, two-week intensive Biogenics training.

PREMENSTRUAL SYNDROME (PMS)

Evaluation

A general medical examination and a pelvic exam are essential, plus intracellular magnesium testing and DHEA.

Therapy

1. Avoid wheat, corn, dairy, citrus, and eggs for two months.

2. Vitamin B6 and minerals, as in carpal tunnel syndrome.

3. Samolinic oil capsules, 1 gram, 9 per day.

4. Biogenics tapes *Balancing Body Feelings* and *Balancing Emotions* 4 times per day.

5. Hypnosis and Past Life Therapy.

6. Build to 75 aerobics points/week.

7. Natural progesterone cream has been reported effective in 83% of cases, although it may take months to find a good regime. Start with one-quarter teaspoon to skin twice a day and build up, if necessary, to one and a half teaspoons. The treatment must begin by the time of ovulation. The cost is $70 to $80 per cycle. Vaginal or rectal suppositories or liquid sublingual capsules are available; use 200 mg. 3 to 4 times per day (may be raised or lowered with symptoms).

8. If DHEA is deficient, replacing it (50 to 100 mg. twice a day) may be more beneficial than progesterone cream.

9. Avoid caffeine in the week before your period.

10. Acupuncture often gives excellent results.

11. Consider two-week intensive Biogenics program at Shealy Institute.

POLYNEUROPATHY

Evaluation

Thyroid profile; folate; B6; B12 (or vitamin profile); essential fatty acids (Meridian Valley Labs); T4/T8 lymphocyte ratio; glycohemoglobin and 12-hour p.c. blood sugar; cancer survey; DHEA.

Therapy

1. B-Complex 100 mg. 3 times per day.

2. Trans-Mins Complete Mineral Formula 3 per day.

3. Samolinic oil capsules, 3 grams, 3 times a day.

4. TENS–intense. May need to place electrodes on body higher than the damage.

5. Acupuncture–regular and intense.

6. Biogenics tapes *Balancing Body Feelings* and *Balancing Emotions* 4 times per day.

7. Stoke the Ring of Fire as outlined earlier.

8. Two-week intensive Biogenics training with Past Life Therapy at the Shealy Institute.

RECTAL AND/OR GENITAL PAIN

Evaluation

Thorough medical evaluation is essential; DHEA; intracellular magnesium testing.

Therapy

1. Be sure to check sacrum rotation. Consider nerve blocks at second and third sacral areas, paraforamenal and paracoccygeal blocks.

2. Intense acupuncture paracoccygeal.

3. Check carefully for depression and treat.

4. Hypnosis and Past Life Therapy.

    5. Two-week intensive Biogenics training if treatment fails.

REFLEX SYMPATHETIC DYSTROPHY (RSD)

Evaluation

This diagnosis is usually made medically. Intracellular magnesium and DHEA are crucial tests.

Therapy

1. Intravenous magnesium up to 15 days.
2. Acupuncture.
3. Temperature biofeedback training.
4. DHEA and Ring of Fire protocol.

SHINGLES

Evaluation

A routine medical evaluation is needed.

Therapy

1. In the first week of the rash, try Acyclovir 200 mg., 1 every 4 hours, 5 times a day, for 10 days.
2. If the Acyclovir doesn't work, consider Flagyl 1 gm. 4 times per day for 5 to 7 days.
3. Intracostal nerve blocks may be useful in the first 2 weeks.

4. Intravenous vitamin C 50 gm. with calcium, magnesium, and B6 daily for 5 days.

5. Intense acupuncture.

If these five approaches don't work, or if the pain persists over 3 weeks after the initial infection/rash, then prompt intervention is indicated.

6. Adenosine monophosphate 25 mg. subcutaneously/intramuscularly daily for 5 days with 1000 mg. of vitamin B12.

7. DHEA evaluation and DHEA/Ring of Fire protocol.

8. Two-week intensive Biogenics program at the Shealy Institute.

THALAMIC PAIN

Evaluation

Thalamic pain may involve an entire half of the body, face to foot. It occurs after some type of stroke. Other than a neurologic examination, DHEA, intracellular magnesium, and amino acid profiles are essential.

Therapy

1. Consider intense acupuncture and TENS ipsilaterally and contralaterally.

2. Otherwise, treat the same as phantom limb pain except for #5.

3. Especially consider Magnesium intravenously,.2 grams per day for 10 days.

4. Cranial Electrical Stimulation and Ring of Fire.

5. Consider a two-week intensive Biogenics program at the Shealy Institute.

VIRAL ILLNESSES

Nutritional Supplementation

For people with acute viral illnesses, such as mononucleosis or hepatitis, the treatment of choice is daily intravenous solutions of the following combination:

500 cc. half normal saline

50 gm. vitamin C

2 gm. magnesium chloride

1 gm. calcium chloride

100 mg. vitamin B6

1 cc. vitamin B complex-100

1 gm. dexpanthenol

1000 units vitamin B12

DHEA orally 1000 mg. per day.

The infusion should be administered gradually over about four hours. This regimen is also powerful for bone pain in metastatic cancer.

CONCLUSION

In closing, I wish to emphasize that the Shealy Institute has specialized in successful and safe alternatives for almost twenty-five years. Our staff is happy to train holistically inclined physicians and health professionals. We provide joint venture cooperation to work with selected physicians in setting up specialized clinics to treat headache, chronic pain, depression, and DHEA deficiency. In addition, Carolyn Myss and I teach Intuition Workshops designed to help you activate your potentials.

The medicine of the twenty-first century is beginning to be available now. Today's miracles will become the standards of the next century. DHEA restoration alone—through our Ring of Fire protocol—should revolutionize medicine worldwide. With the tools outlined in this book, a majority of people can live healthy, productive lives and begin to achieve the optimal human potential of living beyond 100 years of age.

NOTES

1. Len Wyzinski of Georgetown University, unpublished data.

2. Jethro Kloss, *Back to Eden* (Loma Linda, CA: Back to Eden Publishing, 1992).

3. C. Norman Shealy, "Clinical Observation—Vitamin B6 and Other Vitamin Levels in Chronic Pain Patients," *The Clinical Journal of Pain* 2 (1986)3: 203–204.

Bibliography

A Course in Miracles. New York: Foundation for Inner Peace, 1975.

Becker, Robert 0., and Selden, Gary. *The Body Electric.* New York: William Morrow, 1985.

Borysenko, Joan. *Guilt Is the Teacher, Love Is the Lesson.* New York: Warner Books, 1988.

———. *Minding the Body, Mending the Mind.* New York: Bantam Books, 1988.

Buscaglia, Leo F. *Living Loving and Learning.* New York: Fawcett Columbine, 1982.

Clark, Hulda Regher. *The Cure for All Cancers.* San Diego, CA: ProMotion Publishing, 1993.

De Rougemont, Denis. *Love in.the Western.World.* Princeton, NJ: Princeton University Press, 1983.

Feldenkrais, M. *Body and Mature Behavior.* New York: International Universities Press, 1970.

Gordon, Richard. *Great Medical Disasters.* New York: Dorset Press, 1983.

Hamburg, David A. *Healthy People: A Surgeon General's Report on Health Promotion and Disease Prevention.* Bethesda, MD: United States Dept. of Health Education and Welfare, 1979.

Hanh, Thich Nhat. *Peace in Every Step.* New York: Bantam, 1992.

Hudson, Thomson Jay. *The Law of Psychic Phenomena.* Salinas, CA: Hudson-Cohan Publishing Co., 1977.

John-Roger and MaWilliams, Peter. *You Can't Afford the Luxury of a Negative Thought.* Los Angeles: Prelude Press, 1989.

Karagulla, Shafica. *Breakthrough to Creativity.* Los Angeles: Devorss and Company, 1967.

Keen, Sam. *The Passionate Life: Stages of Loving.* San Francisco: Harper and Row, 1983.

Lakhovsky, Georges. *The Secret of Life.* Costa Mesa, CA: Noontide Press, 1988.

Lerner, Harriet Goldhor. *The Dance of Anger.* New York: Harper and Row, 1985.

269

McKeown, Thomas. *The Role of Medicine*. London: Nuffield Provencial Hospitals Trusts, 1976.

Ornstein, Robert, and Swen, Cionis. *The Healing Brain*. New York: Guilford Press, 1990.

Osler, Sir William. *Aequanimitas*. 2nd ed. New York: McGraw Hill, 1932.

Ott, John N. *Light Radiation and You*. Greenwich, CT: Devin-Adair, 1982.

Peck, M. Scott. *The Road Less Traveled*. New York: Simon & Schuster, 1978.

Pelletier, Kenneth R. *Mind as Healer, Mind as Slayer*. New York: Delacorte Press, 1977.

———. *Longevity: Fulfilling Our Biological Potential*. New York: Delacorte Press, 1980

Porter, Garrett and Norris, Patricia A. *Why Me?* Walpold, NH: Stillpoint Publishing, 1985.

Pulos, Lee, and Richman, Gary. *Miracles and Other Realities*. San Francisco: Omega Press, 1990.

Ranke-Heinemann, Uta, *Eunuchs for the Kingdom of Heaven*. New York: Penguin Books, 1991.

Reiser, David E., and Rosen, David H., *Medicine as a Human Experience*. Baltimore, MD: University Park Press, 1984.

Sagan, Leonard A. *The Health of Nations*. New York: Basic Books, 1987.

Salmon, J. Warren. *Alternative Medicines*. New York: Tavistock, 1984.

Sehnert, Keith W. *How to Be Your Own Doctor–Sometimes*. New York: Grosset and Dunlap, 1975.

Seligman, Martin E. P., *Learned Optimism*. New York: Alfred A. Knopf, 1991.

Shealy, C. Norman. *The Self-Healing Workbook: Your Personal Plan for Stress-Free Living*. Rockport, MA: Element Books, 1993.

———. *Third Party Rape: The Conspiracy to Rob You of Health Care*. St. Paul, MN: Galde Press, 1993

Shealy, C. Norman, and Myss, Caroline M. *The Creation of Health*. Walpole, NH: Stillpoint Publishing, 1993.

Siegel, Bernie S. *Love, Medicine, and Miracles*. New York: Harper and Row, 1991.

Smedes, Lewis B. *Forgive and Forget*. New York: Harper and Row, 1984.

Tache, Jean; Selye, Hans; and Day, Stacey B. *Cancer, Stress, and Death*. New York: Plenum Book Co., 1979.

Tart, Charles T. *Waking Up*. Boston: New Science Library, 1986.

Tournier, Paul. *Guilt and Grace*. New York: Harper and Row, 1962.

Index

271